Primitive Expression and Dance Therapy

This book provides a rigorous and comprehensive account of primitive expression in dance therapy, focusing on the use of rhythm and exploring the therapeutic potential inherent in the diverse traditions of popular dance, from tribal shamanic dance to styles such as rock, rap and hip-hop strongly present in our contemporary society.

Drawing on the author's vast experience in the field of dance therapy, the book examines biological, psychological and anthropological foundations of rhythm-based therapies, considering their roots in biological rhythms such as the heartbeat and using such rhythms in therapy. Chapters include:

- The link between human and animal: ethology
- Shamanism
- Gestural symmetry coupling with the other
- Bilateralism as structuring dialogue
- Rhythm dance therapy
- New fields in the application of rhythm dance therapy.

Clinical examples are provided throughout the book to comprehensively demonstrate how rhythm dance therapy can contribute to the use of the arts therapies. It offers a fresh perspective for researchers, psychotherapists and clinicians who want to use dance therapy techniques, as well as arts therapists and those who want to learn more about artistic and cultural dance.

France Schott-Billmann, PhD, is a Psychoanalyst, Dance Therapist and Dance Researcher. She was Program Leader within the Performing Arts section of the Arts Therapy Program at University Paris 5 Descartes in Paris for 20 years until 2011, where she now teaches dance therapy to masters students. She worked with adolescent psychotic patients in the CEREP psychiatric hospital in Paris for 15 years. At present she works at Bellan Hospital in Paris with patients suffering from Parkinson's disease. She teaches in various training programs in Europe and leads workshops all around the globe.

Explorations in Mental Health series

Books in this series:

New Law and Ethics in Mental Health Advance Directives
The convention on the rights of persons with disabilities and the right to choose
Penelope Weller

The Clinician, the Brain, and I
Neuroscientific findings and the subjective self in clinical practice
Tony Schneider

A Psychological Perspective on Joy and Emotional Fulfillment
Chris M. Meadows

Brain Evolution, Language and Psychopathology in Schizophrenia
Edited by Paolo Brambilla and Andrea Marini

Quantitative and Qualitative Methods in Psychotherapy Research
Edited by Wolfgang Lutz and Sarah Knox

Trauma-Informed Care
How neuroscience influences practice
Amanda Evans and Patricia Coccoma

Learning about Emotions in Illness
Integrating psychotherapeutic teaching into medical education
Edited by Peter Shoenberg and Jessica Yakeley

The Philosophy, Theory and Methods of J. L. Moreno
The man who tried to become God
John Nolte

Psychological Approaches to Understanding and Treating Auditory Hallucinations
From theory to therapy
Edited by Mark Hayward, Clara Strauss and Simon McCarthy-Jones

Primitive Expression and Dance Therapy
When dancing heals
France Schott-Billmann

Primitive Expression and Dance Therapy
When dancing heals

France Schott-Billmann
Translated by Terence Holden

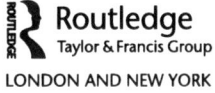

LONDON AND NEW YORK

First published 2015
by Routledge
27 Church Road, Hove, East Sussex, BN3 2FA

and by Routledge
711 Third Avenue, New York, NY 10017

Routledge is an imprint of the Taylor & Francis Group, an informa business

© 2015. F. Schott-Billmann

The right of F. Schott-Billmann to be identified as author of this work has been asserted by her in accordance with sections 77 and 78 of the Copyright, Designs and Patents Act 1988.

All rights reserved. No part of this book may be reprinted or reproduced or utilised in any form or by any electronic, mechanical, or other means, now known or hereafter invented, including photocopying and recording, or in any information storage or retrieval system, without permission in writing from the publishers.

First published in French as *Quand la danse guérit* 2012
by Le Courrier du Livre

Trademark notice: Product or corporate names may be trademarks or registered trademarks, and are used only for identification and explanation without intent to infringe.

British Library Cataloguing in Publication Data
A catalogue record for this book is available from the British Library

Library of Congress Cataloging-in-Publication Data
Schott-Billmann, France
 Primitive expression and dance therapy : when dancing heals / France Schott-Billmann.
  pages cm—(Explorations in mental health)
 1. Creative ability. 2. Dance therapy. I. Title.
 BF408.S3818 2015
 615.8'5155—dc23   2014025517

ISBN: 978-1-138-80471-5 (hbk)
ISBN: 978-1-315-75277-8 (ebk)

Typeset in Galliard
by RefineCatch Limited, Bungay, Suffolk

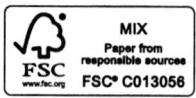

Printed and bound in Great Britain by
TJ International Ltd, Padstow, Cornwall

Contents

List of figures ix
Introduction xi

PART I
Our link to the world 1

1 **Human world unity** 3

   A plural body 4
   Dance and neuroscience 5
   Brain plasticity 7
   The memory of the body 9
   Rhythmic patterns as substitute behaviours 12
   Notes 14

2 **The link between human and animal: ethology** 15

   Mirroring, imitation and simulacra 15
   Non-verbal language 16
   Playing 18
   Rituals 20

3 **Humanisation** 26

   The origin of humanity according to paleontology 26
   The culture, a second world 27
   Note 30

PART II
Traditional dance therapy 31

4 **Dances of trance** 33

   The trance of possession 33
   Therapeutic possession 34

Dances of possession 35
Enthusiasm 38

5 Shamanism   42

Universality and the persistence of shamanism 42
An invisible world 44
The shaman 45
Therapeutic tools 47
The shamanic cure 53
Notes 60

PART III
The humanising process   61

6 The universe of fusion and its dangers   63

The permeable body 63
Primary narcissism 64
Body image 67
Psychosis 71
Autism 73
Note 73

7 Between two   74

Intermediary space 74
Transitional creativity 78
Repetition in rhythm dance therapy 80
Duplication 83

8 Gestural symmetry coupling with the other   87

Symmetry in rites, games and dances 87
The dynamic sources of gestural symmetry 88
The corporeal foundations of gestural symmetry 89
Gestural symmetry in dance 91
Restoring the link 92
Application in the treatment of psychotic and autistic patients 96
The therapeutic treasure of oral cultures: bilateralism 97
Notes 101

9 Bilateralism as structuring dialogue   103

The pair call–reply 103
The calling power of archetypes 105

The pairing of opposites 107
Note 112

10 Symbolisation 113

Descending to the underworld 113
The liberating rhythm 114
Separation from the animal kingdom 116
The 'fort-da' dance 118
The paternal function 120
Notes 128

PART IV
The therapeutic process 129

11 The healing process 131

The creation of meaning 131
Symbolic reorganisation 134
Pacifying, mastering and structuring 137
Sublimation 137
Primitive aesthetics 139
Notes 146

12 Rhythm dance therapy 147

Popular dances for therapeutic mediation 147
Rhythm dance therapy using Primitive Expression 152
Therapeutic tools in Primitive Expression 153
Ethics 158
Notes 160

13 New fields in the application of rhythm dance therapy 161

The social field and dancing for peace 161
Dancing for peace in Israel 162
Clinical applications: neurological disorders 170
Notes 177

Conclusion 179

Bibliography 182
Index 186

Figures

2.1	Ritualised combat between Uca crabs	21
2.2	Traditional ritual hunt of the man-deer (Sardinia)	25
3.1	Dancing women, Paleolithic cave painting, Cogul (Spain)	29
3.2	'The sorcerer', Paleolithic cave painting, the Trois-Frères cave, Ariège	30
4.1	An example of a variety of courtship tarantella dances practiced today	40
5.1	Navajo sand painting	51
6.1	Detail of hell in *The Last Judgment* by Hieronymus Bosch	70
7.1	Drawing by an autistic child aged 9	81
8.1	Cruciform figurine	90
9.1	Yin and Yang	110
10.1	Between image and sign: the marked circle, drawing by a 4-year-old child	117
10.2	The circularity of the call–reply between I and the Other	120
10.3	An initiated unveils the phallus, Villa of the Mysteries, 1st–2nd century BC, Pompeii	121
10.4	Circularity of call–reply between the dancer and the Other	126
11.1	Drawing of a tadpole man by a 4-year-old child	132
11.2	Primitive aesthetics: force and stylisation	139
12.1	The call of the drum: Henri Samba and hailing the Earth	157
12.2	Finding the ancestral gesture	158
13.1	Sharing the rhythm in Jerusalem	168
13.2	Parkinson Dance session with Svetlana Panova	176

Introduction

Our societies have reduced dance to a secondary activity, relegating it to the sphere of entertainment. They have forgotten what the ancients knew: its role in maintaining equilibrium within the individual and society as a whole. Although, today, amateur and collective forms of dance are becoming more popular, too many still consider dance primarily as an activity for single performers or one reserved for women. The old believe that it is for the young; the disabled do not even entertain the notion of participating, imagining a trained and agile body as an indispensable precondition.

Yet dance belongs to everyone.

It was only after a stay in Africa that I was able to appreciate the fuller meaning of dance, beyond its status as a professionalised art performed on a stage before seated spectators, as it has come to be seen today. We can only truly know dance once we have seen everyone dancing in the village squares, whether young, old, lame or disabled, using every means at their disposal.

Such collective dance is an expression of an ancient oral culture, one which, for centuries, was a vital presence in our own western civilisation. It represents, for all peoples of the world, an experience which is musical, somatic, ritual, collective, egalitarian and joyous; a movement uniting all through its common rhythm.

There are so few things which bring us together in our world in which gloom and solitude have become the norm! Finding a response to the perennial question of how we are to live and flourish together today has become all the more urgent. How are we to overcome our fear of the other (the foreigner, the aged, gangs of youths, the excluded, the poor, the disabled, the sick, etc.) without finding a common measure with this other, something shared beyond the horizon of our social and ethnic origins?

Dancing together releases us from our individualism, escaping the boundaries of our self-enclosure and easing our entry into society. It helps us to locate the happy mean between the two poles of our identity: the collective and individual. Dancing puts us into harmony with one another: satisfying our paradoxical desire to say 'us' whilst preserving the 'I', helping us to access the universal without losing sight of the particular.

There exists in dance a universal language embodied by rhythm. It is age-old and speaks to us directly. It allows us to enter into the dance of the other much more quickly than into his spoken language. Dancing enables us to rise above our limitations, de-centreing us from our own petty concerns; it gives us access to a more essential world, a universal of which we are each one the singular expression.

Dance has always played a dual social and therapeutic role. It both fosters group cohesion and has been known for millennia to possess healing properties. In ancient Greece, for example, the dance of the Korybantes treated the illness of the same name, while during the Middle Ages, the dance of St Guy was seen as a means of channelling chorea. It is more commonly known as 'St Vitus' Dance'. There is also the well-known tarantella of Southern Italy, where women working in the fields would dance frenetically when they were bitten by spiders in order to sweat the venom out through their pores. Such ancient techniques of healing through dance are still found in shamanic societies in Siberia, large parts of South East Asia and among the Native Americans. They have also been continuously practised in Africa, where illness is healed through possession dances. These forms of traditional dance therapy all share the characteristics of being group dances accompanied by percussion and singing.

Yet these cultural expressions of social well-being were taken so much for granted that no-one thought to speak of dance therapy until the middle of the twentieth century. The idea of revisiting traditional practices was driven by the anthropologists studying the apparent efficacy of such therapies and their genealogical link to psychoanalysis. For the anthropologist Jean Rouch, inventor of ethno-cinema and the director of a number of films about trance cults in Africa, such techniques amount to a form of psychoanalysis where the couch is the streets.

In Europe, a number of psychoanalysts, such as Jung and Lacan, justified their use by framing them as gestural symbolic representations that were particularly effective in harnessing the emotions. Developments in the human sciences enabled the emergence in Europe of a movement which sought to rehabilitate and give a contemporary character to traditional rhythm dance therapies, bringing them into proximity with modern musical-choreographic sensibilities informed by popular forms of music and urban culture. Among the rhythm dance therapies practised in Europe today, the most widespread form, taught at university level and employed in a number of care institutions, is Primitive Expression. The word 'primitive' here is evidently not to be used in a pejorative sense, rather in the sense of primordial, fundamental, universal. A pedagogical technique focusing on the rhythm-dance interface, Primitive Expression focuses on the rhythmic component and makes use of traditional dances, story telling and singing to bring people together around a healing process which harnesses fundamental rhythms to increase the well-being of participants.

Primitive Expression emerged during the 1950s from the research of Katherine Dunham, an African-American choreographer and anthropologist and a towering figure in American dance (Thorpe, 1990). She studied the Caribbean possession cults, such as Haitian 'vaudoo' which, through possession dances, bring together African divinities and Christian saints to heal sick people by exorcising the god responsible for the illness. Katherine Dunham created the troupe 'Negro Ballet' in 1930. The aesthetic shock produced in spectators by her choreography inspired by the vaudoo dances can be compared to that observed at the start of the twentieth century when 'primitive' objects appeared on the art market, fascinating Gauguin, Picasso and many others by their strangeness, force and presence (Rubin, 1984). Katherine Dunham founded her school in 1933. Here, she fused two musical choreographed American heritages, African and European, incorporating elements of western classical dance and popular dance. Situated between primitive tradition and modern primitivism, such a synthesis required a rigorous deconstruction as a preliminary to bringing out elementary unities at the level of movement. The latter are then organised according to symmetrical couples and supported by a strong rhythm played on the drum. They draw in space stylised, powerful, repetitive and vocalised gestures. It was in 1970 that I discovered Primitive Expression at the American Centre in Paris. The very physical dance was taught by Herns Duplan, a Haitian dancer who had both worked with and been inspired by Dunham's technique. I received my training from Duplan and subsequently have spent much of my career exploring the therapeutic potential of this dance. Although well aware that dance has therapeutic effects, neither Dunham nor Herns Duplan called what they were doing dance therapy. They are thought of as teachers or social activists, but above all, as performing artists.

Marian Chace, a contemporary of Dunham's, was one of the first dance therapists in America. Acting intuitively on the basis of her own experiences, she regarded as self-evident the fact that stimulating the body would help the sick. Today, however, theoretical engagement has become essential, given the demands on dance therapy to treat diverse populations in a variety of contexts such as:

- medical (psychiatric, somatic or psychosomatic problems);
- pedagogical (maladjusted or mistreated children and adolescents);
- medico-social (aged or handicapped persons);
- social (the disadvantaged, incarcerated, excluded and marginalised) and political (ethnic or religious conflicts); and
- personal development (intra-psychic, interpersonal and existential conflict).

Today in Europe, two main currents of dance therapy, dance movement therapy and rhythm dance therapy, are meeting the increasing demand within professional care institutions. Practitioners must be prepared to respond to a growing diversity of needs and to possess knowledge of the conditions governing good practice and therapeutic efficacy.

Crucially, they must be able to respond to the question concerning what types of dance to be employed, since not all are therapeutic. There are certain dances which are destructive, toxic or otherwise unhealthy for the body and mind, leading dancers to focus solely on themselves. Others are somewhat insipid and do not engage the body in any meaningful way. Others, still, are too cerebral, awakening the intellect while leaving the senses and the vital drives unmoved.

The quality of the relation of the dance therapist to his patients is also at the heart of the process. Experience shows us that it is not enough to know how to dance or to teach dance for this process to be triggered. The personality of the therapist, what he expresses of his inner being during a session, and his interaction with the patient, are just as important as the technique employed.

Such questions have been the subject of extensive debate within the domain, a debate which has served both to deepen communication between colleagues and to gain greater recognition for the profession. What is still lacking, however, is a unified language capable of bringing coherence to the research conducted today in the most varied domains, and of creating a common set of references allowing candidates to the profession to compare the number of programs provided, growing in step with increasing demand, in diverse training centres within both the public and private sphere.

It is with this goal in mind that the present book was written, re-edited, translated into Greek, Italian and now English. It is a work informed by several years of clinical experience. As a psychotherapist I have treated a number of disorders through dance therapy, whose mechanisms I will attempt to explain. The book also seeks to place such disorders within a holistic perspective. Mental illness can only be understood within the wider concept of the human personality, one which takes into account both its physical and mental aspects, and which has been formed across the history and prehistory (transgenerational memory) of the individual, and indeed, of humanity as a whole. Neither can we exclude the social dimension: the human subject must be understood in relation to his mother, his parents, others and indeed to his own self. The functioning of the human personality takes place across a series of levels which we must not isolate artificially. It is, therefore, impossible to understand the human psyche without embedding it within an anthropological perspective (i.e. a general concept of man and his cultural production).

Dance is an activity which, within the western world, is placed in the category of the arts. We must, therefore, address the question of art as well as its role within the psychic life of the individual in order to take account of the therapeutic power of dance. The dance therapist must, by definition, study dance together with psychology, which of course, enables him to design programs specifically adapted to different pathologies. In addition, however, the particular character of artistic intervention set apart from verbal psychotherapy must be taken into account. We must also be able to bracket the domain of psychology and examine methods of healing which appeal to other perspectives, such as the shamanism prevalent in cultures distant from our own in time and space. This will allow us to escape the limitations of our ethnocentric thought. We must accept that familiar notions of illness are not the only valid ones, and seek inspiration from methods, foreign to our way of thinking, which have decisively proven their efficacy.

The reader is, therefore, invited to embark on both a geographic and interdisciplinary voyage, which will take us through the domains of biology, paleontology, ethnology, as well as the popular traditions, arts (music, poetry, dance) and traditional therapies inseparable from the religious beliefs of societies.

This multi-dimensional approach aims to shed light in anthropological (which is to say in neither mystical nor psychological nor biomedical) terms on the mechanisms these techniques employ towards the transformation of the person and submit new hypotheses for the approval of those individuals – whether psychotherapist, anthropologist, dance therapist or interested reader – who wish to apply them concretely to the test of their own experience.

Through our research into the anthropological foundations of dance therapy, we hope to contribute to the construction of a more rigorous theory, one firmly rooted in the clinical experience underlying this work. The reader who is interested, from whatever perspective, in the effects of dance will find in this work an engagement with theoretical foundations supported by examples and case studies. Ultimately, however, this work is addressed to all those who feel today, more than ever, the need to understand themselves in terms of the deepest roots of their humanity.

I would like to express my profound gratitude to all those colleagues and collaborators who offered their aid in re-editing this book and contributed to its enrichment:

Natale Spineto, Professor of Anthropology at the University of Turin (Italy)
Patricia Raccah, Teacher specialising in handicapped children, based in France
Jean-Yves Collart, Music and dance therapist, based in France
Ayelet Ranen, Dance therapist, based in Israel
Eleanor Hendriks, Psycholinguist and dance therapist, based in Canada
Annaïk Fève, Neurologist at the Bellan Hospital in Paris
Marie-Hélène Delavaud-Roux, University of West Brittany (Brest, France).

Part I
Our link to the world

1 Human world unity

Insofar as dance appeals holistically to the different strata constitutive of human existence, it represents a particularly effective means of integrating these strata and of organising this existence towards coherent activity. Do we not dance with our body and our soul, our emotions and our reason, our unconscious and consciousness? Dancing allows us to synergise all those levels which make us who we are, yet which appear too often in isolation. We are the inheritors of the dualism of western thought, cut off from others and cut in two: the spirit on one side, the body on the other. There are, however, non-dualist cultures whose way of life and philosophy fascinate the West – a fascination often motivated by nostalgia.

We should, of course, remember that the West also harbours non-dualistic and holistic modes of thoughts resistant to the inhuman dissection resulting from an excessive rationalism attributed wrongly to the unfortunate Descartes (Damasio, 1995).[1] The non-dualist position is present in art, oral culture and in the work of certain philosophers, as well as in the experience of the psychoanalytical cure, where the patient discovers that his own words are capable of liberating him from physical disorders. Freud was one of the first 'explorers of the human soul' to discover psycho-corporeal unity through the clinical treatment of hysterical patients, whose symptoms presented psychic distress 'converted' into corporeal ailments.

It is time to free ourselves from this 'Cartesian' heritage which divides man between thought as the foundation of his existence ('I think therefore I am'), and the body. Freud's message, announcing unmistakably the unity of the organism, is of a 'holistic' character. It is, in this sense, one shared by Nietzsche and could be illustrated by the profession of faith of Zarathustra (Nietzsche, 2003) ('I am only body and nothing more; and soul is merely a word for something in the body').[2]

Yet, he is in equal agreement with the phenomenological current of contemporary philosophy, as well as with the conclusions of the human sciences: the human being is an integrated whole, his mind intimately linked to his body and everything inherited genetically from nature, as well as everything which has marked him socially through culture. Permeated by these different forces, he is a 'being in the world' and can in no way isolate himself from it or from his body.

We might note here that the human being of traditional societies does not have a body, in the sense of possessing it. He is his body, deeply bound with the cosmos, to nature and to his community. In the West, however, dualism persists, enclosing the human subject within an individualist position of isolation and mastery, a position whose alienating effects many have denounced (Le Breton, 1990: 13–28).

Recent advances in the exploration of the biological foundations of the human psyche work in parallel with anthropology to show that the identity of the human subject is holistic and non-dualist, the product of a continuity between body and world. This is a continuity which, as I will now seek to demonstrate, dance is in a good position both to create and to restore.

A plural body

Dance plunges its roots into the 'animal body' of the human, whose biological foundations constitute an integral part of its therapeutic efficacy. Dance is, above all, a physical activity, harnessing movements which produce effects of a physiological nature: the circulation of blood, the oxygenation of the organs, the repairing of the joints and the heart and other stimulating or relaxing effects. To the extent that we may distinguish it from the other levels which constitute human existence, the physical level is the first to benefit from the dynamising effects of dance.

Dance awakens motor functions which register and (re)produce gestural forms and rhythms originating in biologically inherited organic structures of a genetic or neurological nature. It links us to the memory of our species, the phylogenetic traces of which govern programmed behaviour written into the functioning of our bodies: attack, flight, seduction, protection, domination, submission, nourishment, grooming, etc. Inflected from their initial function to the ends of communication, our genetically programmed modes of behaviour serve as the substratum for an archaic motor language found in the animal but equally in the human, either accompanying speech (via hand gestures, facial expressions and postures) or replacing it (in the pantomime of the child, the gestural component of sign language).

Enabling this primordial language to express itself through the motor functions employed in dance gives us access to fundamental and universal neuropsychic forms, an 'unconscious stock' (J.-P. Changeux) of veritable anthropological structures, the malfunctioning of which results in diverse troubles, yet which inversely can be harnessed to remarkable effect in the maintaining and re-establishing of equilibrium. Dance therapy, by 'activating' these structures, putting them into shared resonance and expressing them through gesture, is a particularly potent therapeutic tool.

To be added to this first layer of the 'animal body' is a second, made up of social signs (greetings, gestures, rituals) which stamp it with the seal of culture. Social discourse superimposes itself over our corporeal collective 'archetypal' language. It thereby provides a framework for more individualised forms of expression, which produce, in turn, the third level of personal lived experience. Dance, in other words, constitutes a language in its own right, carrying in similar fashion to words the potently therapeutic capacity for symbolisation. Dance therapy must discover how to make use of this capacity to be effective.

We must not stop at this linking of the human being to its biological-social roots and its self-expression through corporeal language. Dance operates at a fourth level, that of aesthetics, which it shares with the other arts. The search for the beautiful sets in motion the dynamic of sublimation which, in therapeutic terms, constitutes an extremely effective physic mechanism. The spiritual dimension also operates at this level, giving access to the sacred.

Dance and neuroscience

A consideration of some recent advances in neurosciences will be of great use in helping us to avoid the dualism which would make of dance an activity of the 'body' set apart from the 'mind'.

The brain is not opposed to the body

When we dance with our feet we also dance with our brain, the substrate to which the human psyche is directly linked. This is because the brain does not govern the intellect alone. Neuroscience shows how erroneous it is to see in this organ the fortress of the 'mental' dimension. Managing our senses through the sensorial cortex and our muscular responses through the motor cortex, it links them via associative zones and puts us in relation with the world which we 'mime' and incorporate thanks to mirror neurons, discovered recently by Riszolatti (Riszolatti, 2007) and his team at the University of Parma in Italy.[3] These neurons project a representation of the action, whether this has taken place or not. This means that to understand what the other is doing, a subject must activate his own motor neurons which under different circumstances will perform the same action as the one in this case observed. These are the neurons which underlie inter-human relationships insofar as they enable us to identify the other and to understand him or her empathetically (Preston and de Waal, 2002: 25, 1–72).

The brain, thereby, mediates outside and inside without any separation between body and mind, rather in an entanglement of functions. Multiple connections and relays unite different zones of the brain developed successively over the course of evolution. These zones are actively involved in dance.

The hypothalamus

The hypothalamus is 'the brain of the instincts'. Small in size, it is composed of a series of nuclei located in the forebrain. It is these nuclei which induce the states of motivation which lead us to want to drink, eat, make love, sleep, move and so on. The pleasure engendered by such activities resides in the 'pleasure centres' located in these hypothalamic nuclei.

The limbic brain

This is the 'brain of the emotions'. It resides in the 'old cortex', the primitive zone of the brain (olfactory bulbs, hippocampus, septum, amygdale) and controls affective modes of behaviour. Damage to these zones results in serious emotional issues such as anxiety, anger and terror.

The neocortex

This is the wall of the cerebral hemisphere. It is made up of a grey substance which is particularly developed among mammals and constitutes the most recent cerebral formation. We customarily associate it with intelligence. Might, therefore, the neocortex represent the pole of the 'mind', in opposition to the 'brain of the body' (i.e. the hypothalamus), which regulates our instincts, and the limbic brain, which regulates our emotional life? Once again we will have to renounce such a dualism, absent within neuroscience.

In the cortex we find not only concepts but also images, along with the subjective and decidedly corporeal impressions which stir them, or which they engender. The cortex is as much the locus of the senses (insofar as it structures the lived experience) as abstract reason: a musician or dancer uses his 'head' no less than a mathematician does, and we know today that emotion is constitutive of intelligence (Damasio, 2003).

Rhythm and trance

Nerve tissue governs our relationship to the world. Each one of our three billion neurons exhibits spontaneous electrical activity, rhythmic surges which serve to code information coming from outside. Rhythm serves as the key to the translation of these messages: a 'dance of neurons' producing a language for the brain to interpret. These rhythms give birth to cerebral waves and researchers have shown that our perception of beat, as well as our capacity to move in synchrony with it, is a spontaneous aptitude due to the fashion in which neurons are trained to pulse periodically to its frequency (Nozaradan, 2011). This effect serves to link together distant cortical zones (e.g. the auditory and motor zones), creating an immediate motor response to music. It might also be the case that the resonating together of populations of neurons with the musical rhythms (in particular those of percussion) represents a mechanism for the beginning of the trance-like state (Neher, 1962). As such, we could see this state as the product of a synchronisation of musical, muscular and cerebral rhythms and as an intensification of the connections between the two hemispheres (Aquili, 1979). Such a coordinated activation and bringing into phase of 'assemblies of neurons' lead towards the unification of the body through the synchrony of its different parts.

Emotions and ecstasy

The transmission of the nerve signal occurs via the 'neurotransmitters', chemical substances which exist in a variety of forms. The enkephalins, secreted in abundance during repetitive and highly oxygenated ('aerobic') physical activity, create a state of exhilaration. In rhythm dance therapy, as we shall see below, repeated rhythmic gestures intensify pleasure and the secretion of dopamine which is crucial to the treatment of Parkinson's disease. The feeling of joy, an integral element in popular dance, therefore plays an important therapeutic role. The enkephalins contribute to creating a 'modified state of consciousness' which might, depending on its intensity, correspond to trance, ecstasy, or to use a term less foreign to the West, enthusiasm.

Dance is a vector in the reunification of body and mind. It is an activity which is capable, as we see in particular through ritual dance, of using cerebral properties to link inside and outside, self and world through the intermediary of rhythm. We shall see below that this process of linking constitutes an essential element in rhythm dance therapy.

Brain plasticity

In the brain, nothing is definitive or exclusive. It is a highly plastic organ, forever learning and undergoing modification. This endows it with a property essential to therapy, since it follows that one can always hope to induce changes: replace nervous circuits which have been interrupted, relearn forgotten modes of behaviour, and so on.

Epigenesis

The brain is in need of the exterior world for the very process of its development. Although it possesses along with other organs (e.g. liver, kidneys, lungs) an endogenous mechanism, a genetic programme which fixes its stages of development, it can complete itself only via interaction with the outside. The exterior world plays a crucial role in organising the brain, through a mechanism known as 'epigenesis' involving a call–reply dynamic between external stimuli and the brain. The plasticity of the brain has important consequences:

- Man is not only the animal which possesses the longest period of learning, he is also the one who retains it the longest, one might say until the end of his life. He possesses indeed, like the embryo, the privilege of creating fresh synapses and new networks: in short of conserving, when stimulated within a situation of learning, a brain which is 'always young'. It is crucial to 'nourish' the brain by keeping it alive and making it work 'epigenetically'.
- Learning, essential for the brain if it is to develop epigenetically, consists as much in getting rid of useless branches as in creating new ones. According to J.P. Changeux, 'learning is eliminating' (Changeux, 2003: 304). Whenever

we learn, something is organised out of chaos, from the 'noise' of innumerable unorganised synapses. The model to be integrated via learning creates and, through subsequent repetitions, reinforces certain connections. Thus the action learned is never perfectly repeated, as the neurobiologist Gerard Edelman, Nobel Prize winner in 1972, stresses (*Revue Actuel*, 1990). The repetitive gesture, which is characteristic of tribal dances and in rhythm dance therapy, is an example of this mechanism of progressive 'pruning' in the evolution from initially confused and disordered imitation towards purification and ever-refined stylisation. Primitive Expression is often used with people suffering from Parkinson's disease or Alzheimer's.

Coupled movements

Dances originating in Africa have aroused the curiosity of Europeans, ever since they arrived on our shores at the start of the twentieth century due to their energy and the manner in which this is invested in the body. Indeed, these dances closely follow the organisation of the latter, beating like the heart and surging rhythmically like respiration. They do this through symmetrical forms and paired movements, which we discuss at length below (Schott-Billmann, 1989). These structures (e.g. raising the right hand then the left) translate into motor functions, into space and time, the bilateral symmetry of the human body. Moreover, they also express the bipolar fundamental structure of the human being, the binary semantic oppositions outlined by Claude Lévi-Strauss in his study of Ameroindian mythology (Lévi-Strauss, 1990). The Lévi-Strauss paradigm could indeed be applied to other dances constructed around coupled movements to the extent that they are capable, in similar fashion to myth, of awakening (and entering into resonance with) the binary code written biologically into the functioning of the central nervous system. We could, therefore, advance the idea, in taking up Lévi-Strauss once more for our own purposes, that the oppositions present in the movements 'lend themselves to binary oppositions since these are inherent in the mechanisms forged by nature to permit the exercise of language and thought'. We shall allow ourselves, in any case, the homology between the binary opposition encoded in equal measure into the human body, the psyche and social structures, and the coupled structure of the movement of dance. We could, indeed, extend this homology to the music and dance of oral cultures in general. The acoustic coupling endows music and dance with an oscillating movement which finds its echo in the one who listens, reproducing its dynamic as much in the peasant dances of old as in new oral styles represented by the rap of the suburbs. Let us finally note that we must not confuse binary form (i.e. bipolar, or swaying) with 'binary rhythm' which means double rhythm.

Incorporating forms, resonance and reorganisation

Might we not consider the art of an epoch or society as a selection of the forms of highest therapeutic value, and by virtue of this fact conserved and transmitted?

From this perspective, the repetition of the gesture, which is characteristic of popular dance, serves the function of encoding the gesture into the functioning of the body. If, therefore, it is an inherently beneficial form, its effects will be all the more consolidated by such repetition. It is in the interest of art therapy to bring out the therapeutic value of art, not only as 'ex-pression' but also 'im-pression': the reception of sensations (which constitutes the most immediate sense of the word 'aesthetic') and the interiorising and embedding of its forms within the subject. It is in this way that traditional forms of therapy take effect (see Chapter 5), and we can draw on a wealth of anthropological observation to show such effectiveness. Likewise art, in a process analogous to that of learning, exposes us 'epigenetically' to forms proposed by the exterior world, forms which thereby awaken pre-existing structures, entering into phase with them and eliciting an emotional response. This response, bearing witness to our openness to the exterior, initiates a transformation which is all the more accentuated by its repetition. The forms we recognise as 'aesthetic' are those which are capable of inducing the bodily and emotional resonance that we wish to reproduce.

As such, the neurosciences, the arts, therapy and pedagogy consist in the reorganisation of the brain rendered possible by virtue of its plasticity. 'If we one day possess the ability to visualise certain of these entire networks, via new technologies in medical imagery for example, we will perhaps be able to see, in the course of the therapeutic process, the modification of certain networks and the untying of certain "knots" which we might call "neurotic knots"' (Prochiantz, 1989: 80).

We expect of modern rhythm dance therapy the same result, as we would of traditional collective and festive forms.

The memory of the body

Genes are transmitted from generation to generation. They programme the form, place and function of the organs, the stages of development as well as the innate modes of behaviour, attitudes and character traits.

Our genes are the carriers of very ancient characteristics passed from one generation to the next and which have their origins in the pre-human. They carry the marks of evolution, beginning with unicellular, microscopic beings and continuing up to the development of our own species through the play of genetic mutations which we know, since Darwin, are selected according to the advantages they offer.

According to a theory adopted by Freud and still held today, 'ontogenesis recapitulates phylogenesis'. Our brain retains 'reptilian' traces and, as we shall see, we share with the apes a number of genetically coded forms of behaviour. The human embryo retraces, moreover, during gestation, the principal stages of evolution, passing through fish and amphibian phases. It is also entirely possible that the child recapitulates during the course of his psychic development the history of humanity. For example, the 'mentality' of the child, which is so different from that of an adult by virtue of its playful and imaginative character, its intense and corporeal relation to the world and its fascination with rhythmic, homophonic and poetic associations, might simply be the persistence of the mentality of primitive man. We are unable to prove such a theory as our distant ancestors have left far too few traces to permit such a comparison. Yet the fantasy of the 'primitive man', the good or bad savage, dwelling in intimacy with the animal world and nature, continues to live in our imagination which, in essence, still remains secretly animist, just as it still lives in the 'shamanic' world which we shall explore later.

In phylogenetic terms, it was hitherto common to relegate primitive societies of our own time to the infancy of humanity, to envisage them as the children of prelogical thought. While such a position has long been shown to be untenable, it nonetheless remains true that in the mental functioning of 'primitive thought' among the tribal people we call 'primitive', the adult retains a certain childlike, artistic and poetic character, a character which should not be limited to childhood.

Genetic modes of behaviour

The study of genes shows the fashion in which they govern certain of our modes of behaviour, specifically those corresponding to hereditary motor functions. This includes not only reflexes, but also more complex sequences of movements fixed in advance and linked to survival. Pre-established programmes structure actions linked to self-preservation and the preservation of the species. Genes carry the 'moulds' of these types of behaviour, the patterns governing genetically programmed movements and the representations which trigger stimuli.

Animals

All living beings present certain modes of stereotypical behaviour for feeding, coupling, fighting, grooming and child-rearing, each one of which emerges from the integration of partial modes of behaviour:

- combat: this implies the action of biting, threatening and chasing;
- courting: this consists of 'dancing' (undulating), shaking, touching, leading, fertilising the female;
- building the nest: this requires digging, gathering, foraging; and
- parenting: this involves ventilating and protecting the eggs.

None of these modes of behaviour are acquired; rather they are genetically programmed.

Man

Genetically programmed modes of behaviour exist in man in the forms of 'instincts' which do not need to be learned: distancing oneself from danger (e.g. from fire), protecting oneself, searching for food. The newborn knows instinctively how to suck on its mother's teat, an action which involves a complex coordination between different types of actions such as inhaling, imbibing, and exhaling. Such modes of behaviour follow a sequence which obeys a certain rhythm and is determined by its genetic mould, one which compels the body. Programmed modes of behaviour constitute the heritage of our evolution in the form of a latent corporeal memory, which our phylogenetic heritage conserves in its entirety and which can always be reactivated. Indeed, the modes of behaviour acquired through learning will always willingly subordinate themselves before the requirements of such genetic programmes. They are never lost or forgotten and are always ready to resurface given favourable circumstances: states in which conscious inhibitions are relaxed (e.g. in dreams where they are lived fantastically) and certain ritualised occasions where they are invoked while being neutralised of their potential danger (i.e. in theatre or dance).

The recognition of the existence of these genetic structures has modified our understanding of psychic problems, leading us to consider new ways of treating them. That recent research, for example, demonstrates the need to discharge somatic anxiety via the motor system is of particular interest to dance therapy. Indeed, our sedentary existence is a prime generator of somatic anxiety, something which could be addressed through pre-established mechanisms of release.

The discoveries of genetics allow us, perhaps, to explain the universality of certain modes of action and representation which appear to be independent of individual biography. The existence of an innate inventory common to all members of the human race could clarify, for example, the notion of the 'collective unconsciousness' and of the 'archetype' of Jung, as well as the 'original fantasies' and 'primitive scene' of Freud. Such phenomena could be envisaged from the perspective of genetics as the traces left over the course of our evolution, inducing representations linked to hereditary modes of behaviour which are common to all humanity: in short, to anthropological structures of genetic origin.

Programming and creating

Yet the more a species evolves, the weaker its programmed modes of behaviour, which gives way to the possibility of innovation. With the higher mammals, fixed and pre-determined modes of behaviour exist dialectically alongside new forms. We could say that for these species, liberty is genetically programmed: exploratory behaviour and epigenesis are vital to the species. 'Adventurousness' co-exists with pre-determined modes; their harmony creates the necessary balance between security and risk. We are all like the young monkey caught between the desire to hang on to his mother's fur and the necessity to leave it behind to satisfy the drive to explore (Anzieu, 1985: 22–23).

We find in dance a trace of this opposition between two forms of activity: codified gestures and improvised production. The former are learnt, the latter are spontaneous. Yet we should not draw this distinction too sharply: genetics forces us to reconsider our concept of learning by showing the extent to which it is bound with the notion of 'heritage'. Do not the genetic constructs of pre-established modes of behaviour resonate with those 'models' received from the outside world, models which allow these modes to express themselves through forms which they recognise and adopt all the more readily in that they resemble those they are programmed to realise? These exterior models function as potent stimuli in the activation of motor functions. We understand how traditional dances, noted for their dynamic and captivating character, do not so much imprint their forms on the organism as take part in an 'encounter' between exterior and the unknown depths of the self through forms selected for their confirmed aptitude to awaken unconscious and unexpected knowledge: a pre-established and implicit *savoir faire* written into our motor capacity. This knowledge takes the form of a series of latent subconscious traces deposited over the course of millennia, a silent corporeal, phylogenetic memory whose internal structures are re-activated via homologous forms proposed by the exterior world.

Dance, in offering this possibility through forms tested and refined across tradition, becomes the vehicle for the revelation of our potential memory and possesses the same function as the dream: to revise our genetic programmes. Yet, at the same time, it awakens the motor component of the traces left in us by our history: reactivating the modes of animal combat, the hunts of prehistoric man, the work gestures of our ancestors and those of our childish games. It allows us not only to feel but to play out this corporeal memory – the inherited part and perhaps indeed the foundation of our unconsciousness. Creation would be, from this perspective the reactivation of these schemas (programmed behaviour) associating with each other to form new combinations (exploratory behaviour).

Rhythmic patterns as substitute behaviours

Insofar as these programmed forms of behaviour are organised into sequences, rhythm constitutes a key factor in their reactivation. We all have experience of such a reactivation. Hearing a rhythm causes us to move our body in some way: tapping our fingers or feet or moving our head; they are all manifestations of the silent and enigmatic memory awakened by this call, to which the body responds with a perceptible muscular reflex.

Does rhythm awaken genetically programmed modes of behaviour by bringing them into phase with itself? What is the source of the particular aptitude for rhythm within the human being? From a biological point of view, rhythm might well be a substitute for programmed behaviour. It is a particularly precious aid for the human child who, alone among the higher mammals, remains for a long time limited by its motor incapacity due to congenital prematurity. However much 'neotenitism' was favourable to our species, we must recognise that the newborn human is the least fortunate of the young of nature. A chick is able pick at seed almost as soon as it hatches; a foal can gallop after a few hours; all animals rapidly learn movement (feeding, control of the sphincter). However, the human baby remains condemned by its motor-neuron immaturity to immobility, powerlessness and dependence. We may thus suppose a link between the initial distress of the child and its aptitude for rhythm. We should remember that it possesses in a still-rough state the genetic modes of behaviour which are rhythmic because they are exhibited in ordered sequences. The child, for its part, displays an immediate interest in a succession of ordered repetitive motifs, in the rhythmic games, such as 'this little piggy . . .' or 'the wheels on the bus . . .' They take enormous delight in listening to such motifs and formulas, almost as if they were actualising these virtual motions and scenarios through such lyrics. Given the child's inability to realise these movements with its immature limbs, might such schemas of motion find their release through rhythm? This would imply a corporeal bond which, although invisible, is still felt in the limbs, perhaps in similar fashion to the 'muscular sympathy' we feel when we are observing dance.

In any case, this type of stimulation is not a source of anxiety because the rhythm offers the possibility of linking excitation to a form. The child branches his internal sensation into external rhythm which acts at the same time as both the manifestation and substitute for the unaccomplished motor capacity. This enables a discharge of tension. Rhythm, whether perceived or produced, would thus be the capacity to appease anxiety caused by what ethologists have identified as 'sensorial motor discordance', the discrepancy between the felt and realisable motor possibilities. It enables us also to escape from certain painful fantasies by creating simulacra of actions, such as flight or combat. We indeed observe amongst animals in a state of stress recourse to pre-established forms of behaviour: rocking from side to side, shaking of the head, leaping up and down, sucking the fingers, pinching or scratching, etc. Such infinitely repeated activities are stereotypes used by animals in captivity to comfort themselves. They are also employed by those who feel annoyed for whatever reason, as in the case of the rhythmic tapping of the driver stuck in a traffic jam. Such actions are perhaps the echoes of modes of behaviour designed to defeat the pathogenic situation.

We cannot yet speak here of expression or therapy, although we are already dealing with a pacification through motor discharge leading to a restoration of equilibrium – in other words, homeostatic regulation.

The genetically programmed forms of behaviour most frequently employed to re-establish equilibrium are those which echo movements acquired from the mother, in particular swaying or rocking. As a substitute for such movements employed also by the ape mother, they can be observed not only by animals in captivity but also by disturbed children, psychotics or children suffering from maternal deprivation, or equally in a temporary and non-pathological way by a baby whose mother is absent, and, finally, by all those in need of reassurance during a moment of anxiety. We balance with one foot on top of the other and execute in more or less ritualised fashion rhythmic activities such as music and dance. Does not 'rock' music and swing dance explicitly echo such swaying and rocking? The increasing importance of rhythmic forms of expression such as 'rock' and 'rap' might indeed represent a spontaneous therapeutic response in the face of modern anxiety. If the isolation induced by rhythm can become harmful to the one who plunges too deeply into it, as is the case with those who are glued to their portable mp3 players for example, it proves its worth within dance therapy which seeks to establish a controlled form of regression, as we seek to do in Primitive Expression.

Notes

1 Excessive rationalism is an injustice made to Descartes, according to Damasio.
2 Frédéric Nietzsche, *Thus Spoke Zarathustra*, 'The Despisers of the Body' (Penguin 1978, IV, (trans.) W. Kaufmann, p. 34).
3 They discovered that neurons from zone F5 of the motor cortex, activated when the macaque performs an action, are equally activated in another macaque observing the former without itself taking any action.

2 The link between human and animal
Ethology

Genetically programmed modes of behaviour take the form of automatic responses to situations perceived by the individual as triggers of stimuli. With the ever-greater complexity which evolution brings, these constructs, without losing their initial function, become the carrier of new meanings. They become, in effect, veritable animal language moulds, which contain and express intentions and messages exchanged between individual representatives of a species. They may indeed lay claim to representing the foundation upon which dance emerged in the human being.

They are regulated by mechanisms whose fascinating discovery is the work of ethology: the science of genetically programmed forms of behaviour. We will outline those which are used in rhythm dance therapy.

Mirroring, imitation and simulacra

The animal is fully immersed in its world. It flows into the environment and other animals. Becoming other is an instinct of which we can observe many examples in the animal kingdom, most obviously as a mechanism of dissimulation designed to deceive a predator or lure a victim. Everyone knows about the chameleon who assumes the colour of its background to escape predators or the stick insect who transforms his body to resemble the tree to which it clings. We know that the mirror function can be precisely located in the brain: the mirror neurons are responsible for mimetic desire: the desire to mime, imitate, 'copy' and identify with the other. They constitute, in other words, the neurological substrate of the inter-human relation.

The shamans imitate the gestures and voices of the animals and numerous of their dances are animal dances, as are those of Afro-American dance as it emerged at the beginning of the twentieth century (grizzly bear, kangaroo hop, turkey trot, foxtrot), and so on. The sacred dances of the polytheist cults are believed to be the dances of the gods: through them, the dancers become the gods.

In traditional popular dance, when dancers sing and perform together, they offer to each other so many sonorous and visual mirrors. Primitive Expression seeks to make this ritual mechanism its own, presenting to the dancer a multi-sensorial mirror which is:

- visual: all dancers dance in unison, thereby becoming the surfaces upon which the mutual reflection of each by all takes place;
- auditory: they sing in chorus, receiving from each other the amplified, magnified echo of their own voices; the vocal mirror is, in essence, magical insofar as, however much it can be intimidating to hear our own voice, it is equally gratifying and unifying to hear that of the chorus knowing that ours is integrated into it and participates in its harmony;
- rhythmic: all follow the same rhythm, which creates between participants a powerful link, the feeling of belonging to a 'community' of those who share a commonality, a community of 'brothers';
- kinesthetic: all participants feel identical sensations, the same tension and relaxation through the joint exercise of opposing muscles or through the linking of high and low pitch sounds produced by the vocal chords;
- coenesthetic: each individual recognises through the other dancer the manifestation of their own sensations of pleasure, shortness of breath, tiredness, or satisfaction in a surmounted difficulty; and
- emotional: the most impressive mirror is that of the joy which spreads on the faces of participants.

Non-verbal language

The non-verbal dimension is a key aspect of our communication. It is rooted in our animal substrate and plays a particularly prominent role in its simulacra function.

Decoys and imprints

In captivity and other stressful situations, the individual takes refuge in motor discharge governed by pre-established modes of behaviour. Their pacifying influence results from a simulacrum effect where the body behaves 'as if' it were being rocked or nourished, 'as if' it were fighting or eating an adversary, etc. Such illusory forms of satisfaction constitute one of the most disconcerting aspects of the animal kingdom, all the more so in that they concern not only actions but also their very objects. The young monkey, for example, can satisfy itself by gripping onto a strip of fur. Although the response is genetically fixed, the stimulus which sets it in motion is much more plastic. It may content itself with a decoy which deceives the animal by offering it an object with similar properties to the original trigger. We can thus imitate and fabricate a 'false' trigger, as in the famous tests carried out on the stickleback. The female of this species of small fish is sensitive to the red stain which the male has on its thorax: in particular with regards to the role it plays in its spectacular 'dance' of seduction. Yet any red fabric can produce the same effect without any reduction of intensity.

The behaviour of an individual is, throughout life, strongly determined by such lures and decoys. The durable character of this 'deceit' is due to the phenomenon of the imprint, genetically predisposed to trigger stimuli at a given period. For example, a child is programmed to respond to the stimuli triggered by the parent who cares for it. Yet the stimulus can function in a completely autonomous fashion, as long as it is presented to the newborn during the sensitive period of its life. The famous experiences of Konrad Lorenz show us that the young ash-coated goose can attach itself as easily to the mother of another species, as a foam ball, a cardboard box or indeed the etiologist himself!

Rhythm and the maternal decoy

For the young mammal, the object must possess 'maternal' characteristics (e.g. warmth and softness (a strip of fur or a quilt)). These become the famous 'transitional objects' of the human baby. Rhythm serves the same function: for the baby monkey, an artificial rocking device is preferred to an immobile substitute for 150 days. Rhythm acts as a 'maternal decoy' at the muscular level via association with the movement of rocking. Research carried out on human children has also demonstrated the existence of such an effect at work at the acoustic level. The foetus, after all, is exposed to the sound of the beating of the maternal heart during the period of gestation. Several experiments by the British ethologist Desmond Morris have confirmed that hearing the rhythm of its mother's beating heart is beneficial to the child (Morris, 2005: 72–74).

In 466 paintings of the Virgin and Child produced over several centuries and chosen as representations of the mother-child relationship, in 373 (or 80%) the head of Jesus leans against the left breast of Mary. Observations made in the USA show that 80% of mothers, whether they are left- or right-handed, hold their child to their left side, whereas they normally carry loads indifferently to the left or right. We must conclude that they are genetically programmed to carry their child so that it can hear their heart beat.

The exposure of groups of newborn children to a recorded heart beat has a manifestly beneficial effect on the sleep and development (measured in terms of weight gain) of these children. Inversely, those newborns deprived of this recording cry more, sleep less and eat less.

These observations are of key importance to rhythm dance therapy. If a recording of the beating of the heart and the movement of rocking function as 'maternal decoys', the music of percussion accompanied by rocking and swaying movements are particularly well placed to approximate this. This ensures that the activity of the dancing results in a profound sense of pleasure, by virtue of its reactivation of the archaic situation – which, in this instance, recalls the comfort of the child being rocked by its mother.

Rhythm and the action decoy

Rhythm is not only an agent of regression; it does not limit itself to simulating and reactivating the maternal link: we should recall its capacity to awaken genetically programmed patterns by resonating with their internal sequences, culminating in a discharge in which excitation is linked to motor forms. Such discharge is crucial to the organism, a 'biological therapy' for somatic anxiety. It also facilitates the creation of simulacra of essential types of action in relation to the exterior world: fleeing, attacking, protecting, giving, taking etc. This constitutes a powerful mechanism for activating, dynamising and empowering, inciting us to act and turning us towards the exterior world. In calling thus on innate motor schemas which discharge under the guise of a simulated rhythmic realisation, it brings dance into being and allocates it a double role:

- The first is pedagogical: to trigger motor schemas and put the body, which is their instrument of action, to work.
- The second is therapeutic: to prevent or assuage troubles linked to the inhibiting of these schemas by linking their anxiety-inducing excitation to a rhythmic form.

Rhythm provides it thus with a container into which it can flow, a release via a substitute mode of behaviour: a pre-symbolisation; a pre- (or rather non-verbal) language which constitutes, as we shall see below, the foundation of the therapeutic operation.

Genetics and etiology help us to understand how dance can use this decoy to its advantage, insofar as rhythm evokes the mother as both the simulacrum of the beating of the heart and the maternal rocking. We will see the extent to which dance is deeply rooted in the body, to which it is indeed located on the interior frontier between human and animal.

Playing

Playing is a modality of action and is universal among humans. It consists of performing an action in such a way as to depart from the conventional meaning or function of the action, to accomplish something else through this action: elsewhere and otherwise (Huizinga, 2012). It is a function which is already present in the animal kingdom. Games also offer simulacra since they consist in pretending (nipping is not biting). They also harness genetic modes of behaviour while diverting them from their initial objective either by 'revising' them for pedagogical reasons (e.g. in the case of the kitten who plays with a ball of wool in a similar way to which it will later play with a mouse), by applying them to new situations or simply by taking pleasure from their functioning. Playing thereby leads us to participate in an infinite repetition of actions: the dog who brings back, without fail, the stick thrown by his master tires less rapidly than the latter from the incessant nature of the activity; the child who throws an object to the ground and delights in seeing his mother pick it up, refuses to listen to her requests to stop, and so on.

The pleasure taken in play cannot be separated from the repetition; this doubles, with each return, the action accomplished in play. The young child repeats 'Ba-Ba-Ba' and other syllables with the utmost delight. Everything happens as if each action were an imitation of the preceding action, producing a repetitive series which leads the child towards an ever-greater exultation. Later, he or she will playfully imitate his mother or others. This imitation brings together different elements in the education of the child, consolidating their transformative effect and heightening the feeling of belonging to the familial group.

For the ape, as for the human, Piaget informs us, play is essential to development by epigenesis because it helps the young mammal to leave behind programmed modes of behaviour, such as gripping, thereby gaining greater autonomy. The mothers take particular care to punish the child who, for too long, prefers to stay clinging to her rather than playing with his peers. When we see the overly protective attitudes of certain human mothers, how can we fail to notice that the higher degree of liberty accorded human behaviour over the fixed codes of the animal, gives freer reign to the neurotic impact of parents on their children? Amongst the apes the structuring role of play is evident. Games are necessary to the equilibrium of the individual ape: they further its development by inciting it to activate modes of behaviour while, at the same time, helping it to find its place in the group. The young ape who keeps himself at a distance from juvenile activities becomes a-social and anti-sexual. Once it becomes an adult, it remains closed in on itself, its arms folded tight around its body. The females that are obliged to copulate despite their lack of sexual desire treat their children as parasites who crawl over their body, attacking and killing them.

Games thus have a pedagogical aspect and function in similar terms to preventative therapy, while possessing over therapy the considerable advantage of being pleasurable – with joyful repetition ever-increasing their effectiveness. Play is genetically programmed into humans who, among the other higher mammals, are alone in continuing to play, indeed in being compelled to continue, far beyond maturity. We represent that strange 'neotenic' species where the adult conserves a number of infantile traits: absence of hair, plasticity of the brain, need for permanent epigenesis and therefore learning and interaction with the exterior world. Far from representing a secondary activity, play corresponds, in this sense, to a vital biological necessity for humans. It is not, therefore, surprising that it can be found in all societies and constitutes not only a pedagogy, but a veritable psychotherapy. Playful activities are essential and whoever is deprived of them runs the risk of serious damage to their psychological health, as stressed by Jacques Nemo: the president of the association Children, Play and Education – EJE.

EJE's role is to establish centres in Gaza for Palestinian infants traumatised by the war. A number of therapists introduced play into their practice – and not just with children in mind. The great psychoanalyst Winnicott regarded it as the basis of the cure: 'Psychotherapy has to do with two people playing together. The corollary of this is that where playing is not possible then the work done by the therapist is directed towards bringing the patient from a state of not being able to play into a state of being able to play' (Winnicott, 2005: 51). Winnicott fully brought out the nobility of the game, too often considered to be useful for children yet otherwise futile in our societies chained to a pragmatic understanding of reality. No less than Freud reminds us of the necessity of harnessing fictionality: '*The opposite* of play is *not* what is *serious*' he tells us '*but* what is real' (Hamayon, 2012: 80). What can be more serious than the child playing with his or her father, mother or teacher at being a baby, cat or locomotive? This is a seriousness in which the player, whether adult or child, is both 'knower and dupe' (Huizinga, 1949: 51).

There are several categories of game: Roger Caillois in his seminal classification distinguished four: those based on competition (*agon*), chance (*alea*), simulacra (*mimicry*), and vertigo (*ilinx*) (Caillois, 1967). Traditional dances are dances of imitation (mimicry) which often imitate peasant activities (sowing, labouring, harvesting) in which dancers imitate each other. Yet the element of vertigo is not excluded from them when dancers waltz or whirl like dervishes; they often lead to the vertigo of trance. It is these aspects of the game which we appropriate in dance therapy.

Finally, we should remember that games require rules, essential to their therapeutic function. To heal we cannot play in any old way: we play with others, particularly in dance, and we are profoundly linked to these others (the therapist and the other participants) through sharing a common code and framework.

Rituals

Where the game is light and playful, the ritual is serious, solemn: 'adult'. It is not free – it aims to obtain effects. The word may impress by its religious connotation, yet it is not entirely determined by it. Ritual is intrinsic to human experience and is rooted in animal behaviour.

Animal rituals

Ethology abounds in examples of animal rituals established on the basis of behavioural schema. Like play, ritual is based on simulacra. This mimetic behaviour deceives the other, making them believe that we are not what we are. It can be found in all stages of the organisation of the animal world up to man. The human is, indeed, particularly fond of appearing to be other than who he or she is and the theatre and carnival give him the perfect opportunity to do this, as does dance, which Pierre Legendre tells us, is driven by the 'passion for being an other'.

Nature also offers us some different examples:

- Among numerous bird species, the female, in order to obtain something from the male, adopts the begging posture of the chick with open beak. This

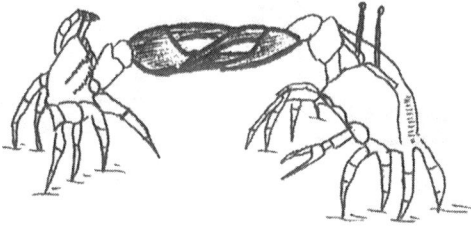

Figure 2.1 Ritualised combat between Uca crabs (large pincer in grey)
Source: J. Huxley

form of behaviour stimulates the male to offer food under the pretext of courtship.
- During courtship, male spiders, instead of eating their prey, offer it to the female. Presenting a gift is, in this instance, a genetically programmed attitude!

Such modes of behaviour can distance themselves considerably from their original form by simplifying, exaggerating and codifying themselves. Huxley cites the case of Uca crabs whose single large claw conveys messages of an extremely varied character (Huxley, 1971). It has developed a veritable coded language through ritualising genetically programmed gestures where the degree of intensity of the threat is communicated through the movement of the pincer (Figure 2.1).

It is generally true of all species that threatening (yet also conquest and courtship) involves the maximum extension of the body, the greatest possible stretching of all limbs, displaying pincers, ruffling feathers, and so on. The reverse, submission (of the defeated or seduced) involves a lowering of the body towards the ground, a contracting of parts, the withdrawing of pincers, the closing of fingers and 'modesty' in appearance: the individual animal 'abases itself'. This universal disposition can be observed in humans when they find themselves before a superior, a police officer, or, indeed, a romantic partner.

The ritualising of genetic modes of behaviour has very possibly been selected and conserved by evolution because of its advantages, on the one hand, for the species, whose losses are reduced (real combat would result in bloodshed) and whose social bonds are reinforced (by shared reference to a common 'language') and, on the other hand, for the individual animal which can employ this mechanism to release tension through an inoffensive motor discharge which remains effective insofar as it is addressed to an adversary who responds to it. The displaying of ritualised substitutes of vital, genetic modes of behaviour possesses, therefore, the double advantage of permitting a discharge and constituting a language. It constitutes a veritable animal language not only for sexuality and combat but also for requesting or welcoming friendship or rejection, territorial claims and identifying the pecking order within a group.

Human rituals

Human rituals possess the function of simulacra. Enacting a mode of behaviour in a codified fashion results in certain effects: it creates emotion and is thought to reach an addressee even if this is an invisible god. For example, in the rituals of the initiation of the vaudoo cult which I observed in Togo, participants intentionally trigger emotional states – fear, suffering, shame, exaltation, pacification – in both the initiate and all those who collectively perform the codified gestures. Ritual also results in the lowering of tension and in the communication of our intentions to the other. Social in character, they begin with a simple gesture of the hand: displaying an empty hand without a weapon, communicates the absence of aggressive intent. Those rituals involving only the individual employ schema such as prayer or the pathological rites of the obsessive who washes his hands 20 times a day or repeatedly checks the state of his apartment. While indeed they may be constraining, these rituals nevertheless have a therapeutic function. As well as enabling motor discharge, they are addressed to an imaginary authority from which the individual seeks to avoid a punishment perceived as merited. They also represent defence (or cancellation) mechanisms. These are effective because they are designed to appease this authority, which in religious rituals takes the form of a supernatural power.

This function of warding off punishment or threat is just as present in religious rites, which frequently involve corporeal schemas of submission to a superior figure (kneeling) and which seek the cancellation of guilt through the repetition of acts of contrition and by proposing sacrifice in place of murder. Religion plays an undeniable therapeutic role (might indeed its decline in the West have been responsible for the rise of psychoanalysis?) as the sum of effective mechanisms for maintaining equilibrium between groups and individuals. Rituals are also present in other traditional activities which possess a therapeutic dimension. To that extent, they aim to transform individuals, inducing them to pass from one state to another (e.g. rites of passage, circumcision, baptism, marriage, burial). Yet they are also carnivals providing an opportunity for both self-transformation and the enacting of transgressive roles rendered inoffensive through displacement from their original function.

Emotional and magical effects

Another function of ritual is to stimulate emotional interaction between participants (Houseman, 2004) and to instil in each a feeling of belonging to the group. It thus plays a crucial role in teaching individuals how to live together peacefully.

The simulacrum is rooted in an expression of the mimetic instinct. The 'copy' harbours a 'magical power' in that it conserves something of the decoy functioning as a double of the real. The simulacrum possesses the capacity to produce effects identical to the model which it 'imitates'. It has the capacity, therefore, to act 'magically' on reality. All sorts of material means are used to perform magical operations: effigies (dolls, the heart of a cow or photographs) are simulacra of the intended person and universally used in sorcery. Yet mimed actions (pricking with a pin or casting spells) are also common. In all cases, it is a question of using the simulacra to 'call', through homology, the concerned person or the action to be directed towards that person. The efficacy of magical action is based on imitation (simulacra) which is the call; magical action is the response of the imitated.

The magic of the simulacrum retains its force for all *homo sapiens*, even the least 'primitive', most rational individuals. A number of politicians and heads of business appeal to it: 'magic, we do not believe in it; but at the same time . . .' The magical object is certainly only an appearance; yet is there also a presence to it? Everything happens as if this were the case. Its effects are tangible, as we have seen with regard to symbolic efficacy.

Man, indeed, invests in the simulacra the very power to raise the dead. Neanderthal man had already used simulacrum for ritualised ends. They placed their dead into the grave in the foetal position, 'as if' they were to undergo gestation and 'as if' the Earth were their mother. We have here a simulacrum harnessing magical effects towards the end of survival after death. Through imitating, or more exactly 'miming', the model allows individuals and groups to solicit and even manipulate it in a certain way. To bring rain, for example, American Indians employ gestures such as clapping the hands and stamping the feet evoking the noise of rain. We can see clearly here that the simulacrum has a function of a 'call' destined to obtain from the thing which is imitated, therefore called 'effects' in 'reply'.

Dance also uses the simulacra to ritual ends. We see this, for example, in the primitive dance of hunters, imitating their animals better to hunt them. The leopard or lion dances are simulacra destined to appropriate qualities of these animals. To behave 'like' the animal allows the dancer to participate in its essence: its flexibility, rapidity, the power of its leaps or the decisiveness of its movements. In this way, the simulacrum maintains continuity with the elements of the universe whose qualities it awakens in the human body.

Art can be considered very much in these terms as a ritual whose goal is to produce magical simulacra. At its origin, it is sacred, inseparable from the search for magical effects. Yet closer to our present day, let us recall that Picasso attributed to tribal sculptures the function of purification whose range he extended to all humans, including westerners. Would we not indeed like to think that the forms recognised as 'beautiful' are 'magically effective' in their ability to transform us?

Whatever the case, there is, in art, the ritual dimension of the simulacrum which causes a metamorphosis to take place 'magically' (i.e. independently of any conscious expression) in the one who enters into contact with it. This power is far from negligible in dance therapy.

The rites which restage mythical scenes offer us doubles of ourselves and our world projected into the supernatural realm in diverse guises whose structure, however, remains constant. The divine archetype of the mother, which has existed since pre-history, is clearly analogical to the human mother. She can be found all over Europe in the form of statues depicting the goddesses of fertility. These universal myths represent our bond to the universal heritage of humanity from its most ancient beginnings. Jung inventoried a number of these primordial common images which he defined as innate schemas of representation and titled 'archetypes': the archetype of the father as that of force, authority, movement, violence, therefore associated with the tempest, storm and war; the archetype of the mother as a figure of softness, nourishment, protection, therefore linked to the mother earth provider, the hearth and the cave. The myth of the hero within this framework would correspond to the experience of the child who has surmounted the ordeal of its initiation into humanity, an ordeal in which play nevertheless constitutes one of the principal stages.

Myths cannot, therefore, be reduced to abstract figures. They make up the common moulds for our representations of divinity, yet are in no way disincarnate. The traditional gods to which polytheist religion attributes distinct domains (god of the sea, god of the underworld, goddess of love, in Madagascar, the thief god of cattle or in the *Bori* cult of Niger, god of conjugal infidelity). These resemble men to such an extent that they become incarnate in human individuals through possession.

Ritualised play, theatre and dance

The simulacra in play consists in executing the same modes of behaviour employed in 'serious' activities, yet with a difference which involves not so much an attenuation as a deflection towards 'another' intention and, importantly, an awareness of this deflection. This is the magical time of the conditional, the time of the simulacra: it is 'as if' the child were a locomotive or a doctor; which it is not . . . yet which nonetheless it is.

The recourse to disguise, face paint and the mask render the simulacra more effective. Might this, as such, be understood as a 'call' to the original to manifest itself 'in response' to the behaviour, emotion and appearance of the player? The simulacrum of the game, in other words, is inseparable from a state of transformation. Let us, therefore, make the most of dance therapy, because it is the 'detour' which enables, under the protection and efficacy of 'pretending', of 'not being serious', to embark for war, express rage or be seductive and tender. It allows us to express a huge variety of sentiments which are truly felt, yet are displayed in such a way as to neutralise them and which, in addition, pass, under the shelter of the veil of the simulacra, the censure of the superego insofar as they are only carried out 'for fun'.

In a number of traditional societies, theatre and dance are also understood as forms of play.

We will take, from numerous possible shamanic examples, the case of the Siberian ceremony recorded by Roberte Hamayon. The shaman here wears a costume made from animal skins and reindeer antlers and then dances while leaping, bellowing, stamping and shaking his head. Meanwhile, the participants, in their gestures and songs, also imitate the animal world 'trotting, stamping or

The link between human and animal: ethology 25

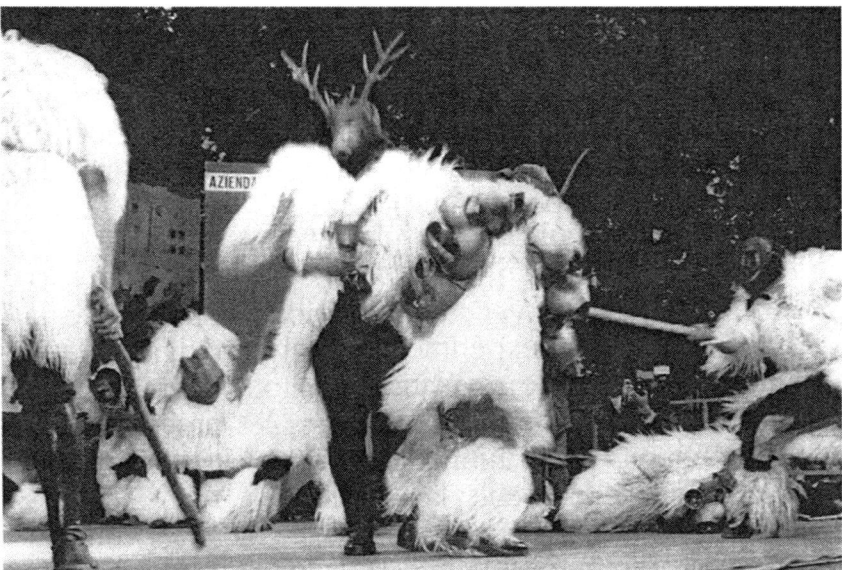

Figure 2.2 Traditional ritual hunt of the man-deer (Sardinia)
Source: Photo by F. Schott-Billmann

leaping in similar fashion to the shaman, and imitating, as he does, the rutting stag. We also find flapping movements of the arms spread out like wings, imitating the great birds in their rites of courtship. The imitation of animals is equally present in the chants which accompany these dances or alternate with them, both in the form of onomatopoeic sounds which evoke the amorous calls of these species and in speech ('let us trot like the elk, let us trot like the reindeer') (Hamayon, 1992: 71).

These ceremonies, which still exist in some parts of the world, give the participant the opportunity to put his own animal nature into phase with those of the animals which surround him. Dance possesses a double role: it binds the dancer in tight bodily relation to his or her corporeal roots; it also enables the expression of potential genetic modes of behaviour, making use of the history of our species as a framework for the more singular expression of our individual history.

3 Humanisation

The gulf between animal and human, for a long time considered too wide to be bridged has, more recently, come to be seen as being considerably more narrow. Biologists, geneticians and ethologists, in establishing the common roots of animal behaviour and certain forms of human behaviour, show that neither communication nor ritual are the exclusive prerogative of the human. They accordingly find themselves in the company of paleontologists who situate the emergence of our species unequivocally in animal societies.

The origin of humanity according to paleontology

To the extent that dance is an awakening of corporeal memory, a re-enactment of the past, a way of connecting to our roots, it enables us to bring the modes of behaviour of our primitive ancestors to expression, those which have left in us the traces of the long 'saga' of the passage from animal to human. Dance carries and unifies within itself the successive strata of this adventure.

Paleontologists were for a long time in agreement that the human species came into existence in Africa following an ecological catastrophe which obliged certain groups of apes to evolve towards humanisation (Morin, 1973). Yet new discoveries about our 'ancestors' in different sites around the world have obliged us to consider other scenarios for the 'birth of man'. We are no longer able to locate the origins of humanity exclusively in Africa, although here, in the absence of other well-established scenarios, we will retain this narrative of origin less in the form of scientific truth than as a myth of origin: in somewhat similar fashion to Freud's speculations on the primitive horde. Both offer a symbolic staging of our beginnings, inciting us to meditate on these while exciting our imagination. Indeed, such an exercise offers rich material for improvisation within masked theatre or dance and I, myself, have employed it to this end on numerous occasions.

Africa is the mythical cradle of humanity. Whether or not we are dealing here with a myth, one fact appears likely: the passage to the upright or bipedal state represents, according to the pre-historian A. Leroi-Gourhan, the decisive step towards humanisation (Leroi-Gourhan, 1985: 2, 135). It is this postural straightening which makes possible the 'unlocking' of the cranium, and therefore the expansion of the brain as well as the liberation of the hand orientated henceforth towards tasks other than locomotion. It could be said that man is intelligent because he has hands, but equally that he has hands because he is intelligent! Life in the Savannah caused the ensemble foot-hand-brain-tool to function in synergy, engendering in the process reflective thought which is the result, according to palaeontologists, of the separation between the intention to act (brain) and its realisation (hand). The tool, prolonging the hand, prolongs also the mind which interacts with it, and becomes thereby a powerful agent of hominisation. It is from this process that language originates, emerging in those valleys surrounded by cliffs, the gorges of the Olduvai in Tanzania, the banks of Lake Turkana in Kenya, where the genealogy of our African ancestors begins. It is dance which harbours within itself the stages of their evolution.

Bidepal motion is recalled by the vertical standing position of popular traditional dance. It is first seen with Australopithecus seven million years ago, the species of Lucy, the famous small hominid who is a distant cousin of Man.

Repetitive rhythms resulting from regular strokes or beats was discovered by *homo habilis* three million years ago. From the regular 'bay leaf' scallop around the edge of their flint blades we can surmise that they worked to rhythmic percussion. Such objects similar to the engraved plaques (*churingas*) of the Australian aborigines very possibly served then as now to beat out rhythm and chant tales (Leroi-Gourhan, 1985, 1: 266).

Homo erectus, emerging on the scene 2 million years ago who, through his mastery of fire 700,000 years ago, marks a decisive step towards humanisation, liberating the nighttime from the insecurities associated with darkness. This encouraged conviviality and collective activities such as dance and singing during times of rest. Great importance has, from the very earliest times, been attached to times of festivity. 'Village places' were reserved for leisure, kept at a distance from activities such as cooking food or making tools (biface, racloir, scraper, etc.).

The capacity for representation, which is, at the beginning, a simulacra of reality comes to us from *homo sapiens*, the founders of our species, who arrived 250,000 years ago, a little after Neanderthal man.[1] They were faced with the last ice age of the quaternary period which continued until 10,000 years ago. Clothed in animal skins and fearless hunters, *homo sapiens sapiens*, our ancestors, first emerged in the rugged guise of the so-called 'Cro-Magnon' man, 35,000 years ago while the glacial period was still very much underway. *Homo sapiens sapiens* distinguish themselves from all who proceeded them by the practices of painting and burial, testifying to a capacity for representation with infinite consequences for the destiny of humanity. He is not only a social animal but an animal who symbolises.

The culture, a second world

The invention of a 'second' symbolic world, expressed through funerary rites with the burial of the dead in foetal position (the simulacra of rebirth), bears witness to a consciousness of death (therefore of time) and the belief in life after death.

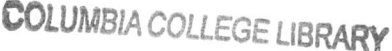

The first graphic forms of representation are around 30,000 years old and are the work of Cro-Magnon man. We are referring here to the cave art of which the Lascaux caves constitute a magnificent example. On their walls we find realistic figures (animals such as bison and horses) alongside abstract forms (grids, crosses, etc.) whose deciphering has still to be accomplished. This 'second world' represents the supernatural powers which *Homo* perceives in nature, materialises in cave paintings or in dance.

This passage from animal nature to human culture took place over millions of years, passing through a number of intermediary states. How, with the lacunas of paleontology, will we ever be able to trace this route? We must renounce such an ambition on the historical level, although myth and art carry its vestiges and show us the mechanism by which it was accomplished. Dance testifies to this link, as does the ritual mask, by superposing the animal, human and divine, one upon the other (Sike, 1998). Culture does not dissociate itself from Nature, but integrates it; the two domains converge in a super-nature, the 'divine'. The dancer is the animal-man-god, an identity inaccessible to everyday reality and which he feels whilst in an 'other', dancing, state (or under a mask). This identity is, however, essential to him, the most profound stratum of his human 'nature', one which endows his artistic practices with their primordial therapeutic foundation.

Dance is the 'body' which 'crosses history' (Nietzsche, 2003: 86). It reawakens the human being at the dawn of the species, allowing successive waves of enthusiasm to rise within us through its playful intensity; through the joy of rediscovering the bonds which link us to both our deepest foundations and to the surrounding world.

It shows us that those elements which render dance therapeutic have been in place since prehistoric times. Dance heals from solitude when it rhythmically links dancers and repairs the rupture between body and mind (by employing spatial terms to express the characteristics of the human body): bidepalism, verticality, the feet rooted to earth-as-nature (the drives), the head inclined towards the sky-culture (the world of symbolic representations) is perhaps the first and most radical line of defence against mental illness. It awakens vital energy through recourse to rhythm and links the dancer to his or her ancestors by reactivating the initial steps towards humanisation and reliving them symbolically. It is, moreover, an inherently aesthetic experience, a particularly effective mechanism which is spontaneously and inherently therapeutic. These conditions endow dance with its therapeutic potency up to the present, remaining ever in force, straddling human history.

Since prehistoric times, the human being has imagined invisible powers at work behind the appearance of things in the world. Deeply animistic, he 'perceives' invisible spirits 'behind' the trees, sources of energy, flowing water and even in objects which seem to us now to be inert, such as stones and rocks. He sees divinities in action in natural phenomena such as thunder and lightning, volcanic activity and earthquakes, but also in regular events such as the diurnal course of the sun, the rotation of the stars and the return of the seasons. Dance represents a potent tool for linking to the supernatural world or voyaging into an invisible

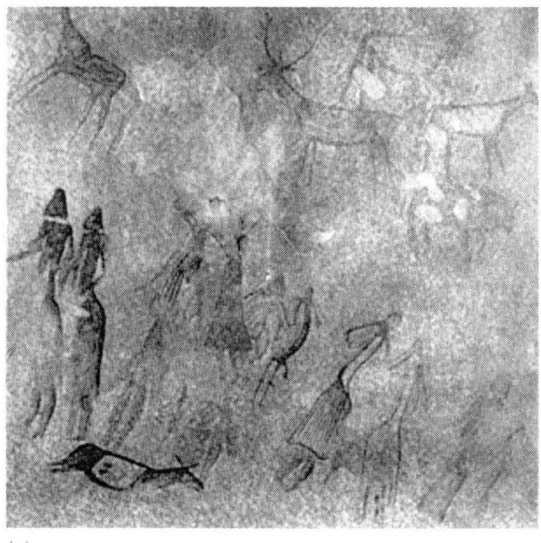

(a)

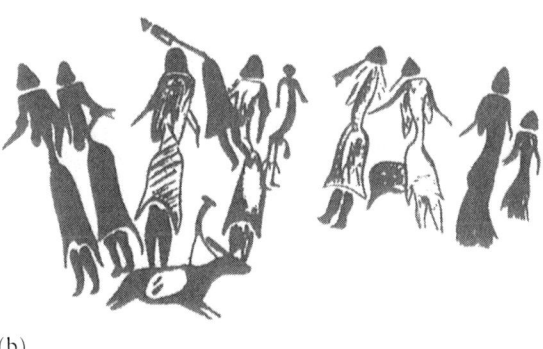

(b)

Figure 3.1 Dancing women, Paleolithic cave painting, Cogul (Spain)

Source: www.persee.fr/web/revues/home/prescript/article/hispa_0007-4640_1991_num_13_1_1686

world because, through its perennial instruments, which are the insistent, rhythmic sound of the drum, repetitive gesture and chant, it induces a state of trance, which serves above all as a means of passage. On the neuro-psychological level, trance is an example of a modified state of consciousness (MSC) profoundly different from our everyday state (Clottes and Lewis-Williams, 1996: 11–28). The subject exists in a second state, plunged into a 'second world' which for Paleolithic societies (yet also for a number of traditional societies today) is the spiritual world, the kingdom of the spirits, of ancestors and divinities. Trance, like the dream and hallucination, is a state of participation in this world, and the person who is in this state draws on its power, energy and healing force (Figure 3.1).

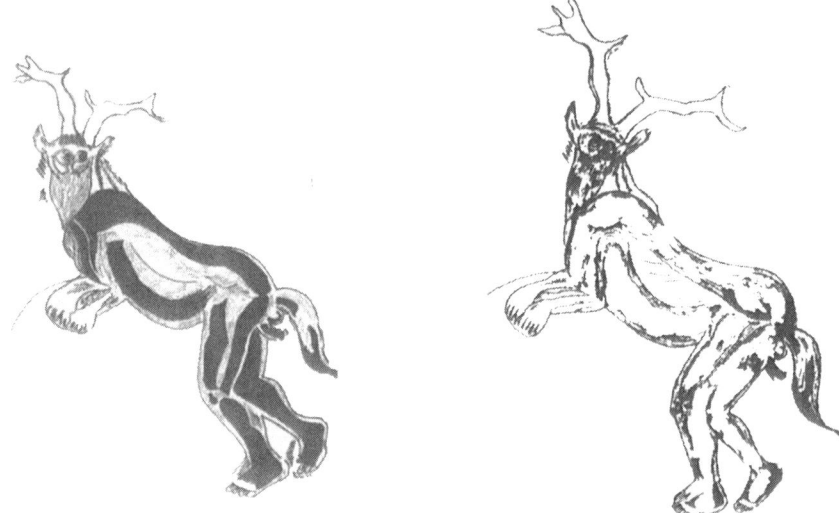

Figure 3.2 'The sorcerer', Paleolithic cave painting, the Trois-Frères cave, Ariège
Source: lecheneparlant.over-blog.com/article-les-monstres-divinities-hybrides-cave

This property of trance has been known since prehistory and the walls of the Magdalenian caves have conserved for almost 15,000 years the evidence of trance states (Bourcier, 1989: 34), which are still practised today as a key element in the rituals of traditional healing (Ruspoli, 1986: 88–89).

A well-known example is the famous 'sorcerer' of the Trois-Frères ('three brother's') cave in the Ariège region of the South of France. Half animal, half man, he resembles the shamans of today who, covered in animal skin and masked, converse with animal spirits to enter a modified state of consciousness (Figure 3.2). He invoked the supernatural forces to enter into the world of men and into his body. Such ancient dynamics remain in force today in the world of shamanism and we will return to them below.

Note

1 They date from 300,000 years earlier and perhaps constitute another species.

Part II
Traditional dance therapy

4 Dances of trance

Thanks to archaeological discoveries we now know that the 'hunter–gatherers', the nomadic cultures of the first human societies, already called on therapeutic trance harnessed by the shamans – those traditional healers whose calling was both artistic and therapeutic. Today, we group together under the name 'shamanism' the ensemble of spiritual and therapeutic practices which have recourse to modified states of conscience: cults of possession practised across Africa, and the shamanic practices which are widespread in Siberia, Asia and America.

The trance of possession

Possession involves metamorphosis, becoming someone else or something other. The body is entirely inhabited by a personality other than that of the familiar self. This self exists in another alienated, 'altered' state: a supernatural being 'descends' into the body of a human who becomes the 'theophany' of this being. The state of possession is a trance in which the supernatural being is a god, a spirit, or an ancestor who speaks through his mouth and makes his body move. In the state of possession, a god 'occupies' the body of the subject who mimes its characteristics before returning to the ordinariness of his habitual existence. He incarnates the 'other' personality which can literally lead to his metamorphosis. Identification can manifest itself not only in the performance but also in the appearance of the dancer. He becomes an ape leaping from branch to branch to the tops of the trees, or adopts the seductive behaviour and lithe gait of the water deity. Yet the approximation to these personas is so radical that we may, on occasion, observe old women temporarily losing their wrinkles and the stiffness of their joints as they become alternatively a mischievous little prince, a seductive young princess, a king full of majesty, an intrepid warrior or a roaring tiger (Schott-Billmann, 1985: 13–14).

The desire to escape the limitations of the self – to become another – constitutes an essential part of human experience; yet possession can be pathological. Before the development of medication capable of counteracting states of delirium, our psychiatric hospitals were full of patients convinced that they were Jesus Christ, Napoleon, or Joan of Arc. Such acts of possession can be observed on all continents, and today still constitute an integral element of social life. They take place publicly during festivals, where an entire group accompanies the sick person as they heal. The involvement of the cure in collective festivities, as the occasion for relaxation and play, is somewhat foreign to the western concept of therapy as an activity executed with sobriety.

Possession has been given a bad press by monotheistic religions where it is considered as emanating from the devil. It is regarded as malevolent: an evil to be exorcised.

Therapeutic possession

From the perspective of the polytheistic religions, sickness is an unfortunate possession, expressing the discontent of a divinity. The possession cults establish a link between the worlds of gods and men. An ensemble of rites allows the shaman to recognise (diagnose) a spirit responsible for the illness, converse with it (through symbolic language) and to exorcise it through theatrical language, using dance, costume and role play. Ritual possession brings the divinity revered by all onto the stage to transform it into an ally, henceforth beneficial and socially valorised. Ritual possession is, accordingly, of great therapeutic efficacy (Schott-Billmann, 1985: 71–99). To incarnate, for example, a god of war enables the subject to exorcise his aggression (i.e. liberate it from its pathogenic character by re-orientating aggression in a positive way, thereby channelling its expression). The state of 'insanity' – the initial disorder – is regulated by dance. We have here a very ancient form of dance therapy whose presence in the Greek Dionysian tradition is made known to us by Plato: 'to dance to the pipe with the help of the Gods to whom they offer acceptable sacrifices, and producing in them a sound mind, which takes the place of their frenzy' (Plato, *The Laws*: VII: 791). Indeed Aristotle reminds us that Bacchic dance and song enabled participants to surmount crises of depression by purging them (catharsis) of their harmful effects (Aristotle, 1959, V: 1342).

According to Jung, our illnesses are caused by the gods whom we have neglected, while Freud saw in the psychoanalytical cure the means of recognising and expressing unconscious desire. For psychoanalysts, the gods are symbolic representations of the drives which we must express if we do not want to fall ill. Psychoanalysis, the possession cult and exorcism envisage here the same object: the capacity of the patient to provide a symbolic release for these psychic forces which appear to emanate from elsewhere, insofar as they are not acknowledged by and integrated into language.

While western societies attribute psychological and psychosomatic disturbances to unresolved, unconscious conflicts, traditional societies consider such mental and physical disturbances (or any series of troubling events) to be the work of a supernatural entity (e.g. the work of a god who has been neglected, an ancestor, a spirit overlooked or hurt by a lack of respect). The illness is a manifestation of the god's displeasure; inversely, making peace with the divinity will trigger a recovery. The efficacy of such divinities resides in their very ambivalence, which permits them to make the subject move from being sick – possessed negatively, to being well – possessed positively. The god gives the sick person beneficial qualities and powers. Psychoanalysis speaks of symbolic reorientation: the re-orienting of the drives towards new non-pathogenic representations. In traditional therapy, healing consists not only of expelling the pathogenic god, but of beneficially re-orientating its forces via the mechanisms of canalisation. Adepts know that, to incite a divinity to 'descend', it is often necessary to begin by 'miming' the dance of possession (i.e. knowingly executing its choreography). Dance, which is at first controlled, becomes, little by little, a trance of possession. The progressive character of this passage from human to divine sometimes creates misunderstanding among certain European ethnologists. Michel Leiris suspected the adepts of the Ethiopian cult of the zârs were attempting to deceive him (Leiris, 1958). Yet, he ignored the fact that it is their practice to call on the gods to incarnate themselves through pre-established forms.

Dances of possession

The traditional practice of 'dance-therapy' through trance is a form of possession dance found in all polytheistic societies. Here, dances of possession are considered to be therapeutic and exorcism is accomplished through a codified choreography. Traditionally, each divinity received its own dance with a strict set of rules to ensure faithful representation. The dance of a god of war looks nothing like that of a goddess of love. The dances of possession thus enable us to experiment with a range of persona, bringing to expression in codified fashion diverse emotions while containing and regulating them through their divine channels.

A possession dance allows the subject to give overt expression to that which dwells within: a force which reconciles itself with those other interior forces which cannot otherwise find expression except through sickness. It bestows upon all these forces a recognised, authorised and valorising language, complemented by the element of pleasure inherent to trance. Possession dance thereby bestows on the emotions a language through which they can express themselves; this constitutes the core of its therapeutic efficacy in traditional societies.

Concretely, healing takes place when a ritual reconciling man and divinity is celebrated before an audience, using the symbolic language of music, theatre and dance. It is by entering into a trance that the possessed comes into contact with the divine world. Called by specific musical devices and hymns, the spirit, recognised and respected, manifests itself positively in the sick person's body. This manifestation consists of a series of coded dance movements, which are also specific to the god and help to identify him (as stated above, the choreography belonging to a war god would be without a doubt very different from that of a sea goddess). One observes this traditional dance therapy at work in both African and Haitian Voodoo rituals, in the Brazilian Candomblé, the Cuban Santería, and in many other ritual dances performed by polytheist forms of spirit worship.

Africa

In Africa, the polytheistic ancestor cults in which trance and possession are practised are far from disappearing. Indeed, since independence, they have gone from strength to strength. Long suppressed by Christian missionaries, they once again enjoy official recognition. The cults of *Vaudoo* in Togo and Bénin, the *Dlo* in the Ivory Coast, *Zebola* in Congo, the *Bwete* in Gabon, the *Bori* in Niger, the *Tromba* in Madagascar (to list only a few) are practised by all sectors of society alongside the great monotheistic religions (Islam and Christianity). There is, in effect, no incompatibility between the monotheist and polytheist vision: the sovereign God can be served at the same time as multiple secondary gods closer to the human world. So close, indeed, that they become incarnate through our bodies: they *possess* us. This aspect of religion has proved more difficult to suppress in Africa than it was for our Celtic ancestors constrained to convert to Christianity and to follow a single God.

To identify the god responsible for the malaise, the African drummer beats out specific rhythms. The fact that one of these rhythms resonates with the body is not enough for healing. A long process is required, one of initiation, which re-orientates the god responsible into a positive and beneficial force, on the condition that it is honoured regularly. The mechanism of this cure involves, as does all therapy, a phase of regression and sacrifice, followed by a process of re-symbolisation which allows the energies of the person who is sick to bring new representations into being (e.g. the god of war or the goddess of love).

In Morocco, the *Gnaouas* deliver their members from illness through intense forms of dance in which participants repeatedly hammer the ground with their feet. It is a rite of possession.

South America

Candomblé is one among a cluster of Afro-Brazilian religions practised in Brazil, as well as neighbouring countries such as Uruguay, Paraguay, Argentina and Venezuela. The gods of Candomblé are invited to enter into the *terreiros* (sacred spaces), incited by music, drums, chants and dances. They show themselves during the ceremony to certain initiates who enter into a state of trance and who then become the intermediaries between gods and men. Today, around 3 million Brazilians are followers of *candomblé* (despite the disapproval of the wealthier classes).

Other countries

In Australia and in China (where Taoist cults of possession can still be found), the arrival of technology has not prevented the traditional healer from using trance and possession dances: therapeutic tools which have been refined over centuries and which are still remarkably effective. A common form of ritualised trance, described in minute detail by ethnographers, is a ritual for spirit possession practised by individuals, even if the event is collectively held. An anthropological reading of these phenomena reveals their social and psychological importance. Indeed, recourse to the divinities permits subjects to symbolise their desire, to articulate conflicting emotions, and to express emotions as psychological forces. Each dance, if not every gesture, opens its own symbolic space, giving a symbolic outlet for effects that were pathogenic due to being poorly symbolised or perhaps not at all. The therapeutic efficacy of trance rituals no longer needs to be proven. One also sees the persistence of these dance forms in our own Christian cultures.

Some ancient Mediterranean trance

The Corybantic dance

In ancient Greece, Corybantes are Cybel's priests and they dance in a state of trance. The Corybantic dance was used for therapy 'to quiet the patient's internal phobia. The corybantic dance could not relieve the external symptoms but could regularize them: it integrated them in a shape of religion.' Dodds states that a corybantic ritual was a musical diagnosis (Dodds, 1977: 103 and n.102). The patient listened to several types of sacred music. Priests studied the patient's reaction identifying thereby the god responsible for their illness. The second part of the ritual would then begin. A sacrifice was offered by the patient to the relevant god, followed by a dance celebrating the pacified god (Delavaud-Roux, 2012).

Some modern Mediterranean trance

The traditional practice of dance therapy, which flourished in the West up to the late Middle Ages, can still be observed in certain regions of Europe. The mythical figure of the spider, considered to be responsible for certain illnesses, is still exorcised in magical religious dances called tarantellas in Puglia in the South of Italy, or in the dances of the *argia* in Sardinia.

The tarantella

The 'taruntula' of the tarantella is a mythical spider. It is said to bite women, causing them to suffer from lethargy. The women are treated using a particular dance – the 'tarantella' – which is played on the violin. This is an exorcism in which dance and music play a central role. The dance creates an intense state of excitement within the women, which ends only at the conclusion of the exorcism carried out collectively by the group (De Martino, 1966). The specialist musicians of the tarantella tradition, who are often blind, not only know the different tarantellas but also the respective spiders to which these are attributed (e.g. mischievousness, childishness, eroticism, bellicosity, etc.). As soon as the patient hears the melody of her spider, it is as if she suddenly recognises what has been dwelling within her without her knowledge. She leaps to her feet and dances – sometimes for three days and nights without stopping – until she is healed.

The argia

This is the local name given to a spider in Sardinia which, for the most part, preys on male Sardinian peasants. Its bite leads to three days of intense pain, abdominal cramps and a profound state of depression, symptoms which are interpreted as the side-effects of possession. The argia incarnates the spirit of a dead person or child (Gallini, 1988). As in the Pulgia region, music and chants serve therapeutically to pacify the pain and anxiety of the victim. The patient or the wider community strive to unmask the spirit responsible for the illness through music and dance.

The Anastenaria

Associated with Saint Constantine and Saint Helen, the Christian heirs of the healing gods of Graeco-Roman antiquity, the *Anastenarides* are members of a mystical and therapeutic cult. Each year they dance over hot coals to exorcise demons and purify themselves (Schott-Billmann, 2006: 169–182). The altered state into which they enter is not that of trance, which involves a loss of consciousness. They are in a state of lucid possession: they know what they are doing, who and where they are: they have been possessed by the spirit of the saints. We call it a 'Mediterranean' trance as it was practised in ancient Greece.

Enthusiasm

It was also called enthusiasm, signifying etymologically, to have the god in oneself (*en-theos*). This 'God' is in fact the Rhythm Dance: an activity which activates and organises enthusiasm (i.e. it enables us to experience a force which takes hold of the body and causes it to leap beyond its habitual limits).

Overwhelmed by the spectacle of the 'negro dances' in Paris in 1925, Phillippe Soupalt wrote: 'I understand everything which separates the conception that we now hold of dance and that of the Negros. We can now no longer understand the force which animates them, which makes them leap and bound' (Soupault, 1986: 38). We no longer understand this force because it is an expression of the exhilarating feeling of vitality and strength which emerges from the link to the cosmos, to the group, to the primitive and ancestral animal heritage we evoked above. We are cut off from this and are reduced to our own energy, which frequently appears to be dramatically reduced among the choreographers of today.

If we want to propose to our contemporaries the joyful experience of a body permeated by a dancing force, we must reconnect to the tradition of enthusiasm, giving birth to new 'intensities' by tapping into the ancient primitive foundation still active in tribal dance. Such is the challenge which Primitive Expression sets itself, recreating a non-religious 'shamanic' ambience through rhythm, the group, the voice, and the dynamism and beauty of movement.

Enthusiasm is the state cultivated by the European peasant dances which celebrate the forces of nature and which can count among their ancestors the dances of ancient Greece. They became our popular dances, which stand out by virtue of their vigour, insistent rhythm and the joy they inspire in the dancers. Peasant dances functioned for centuries as an example of dance therapy, occurring during traditional festivals. These dances, performed by groups to the rhythm of a strong, pulsating beat (which the peasants mark by striking their sabots), took place under the aegis of solar events, solstices, equinoxes and mythological events (e.g. Candlemas on 2 February, the cult of the dead on 1 November, the feast of all saints). They possessed all the characteristics – rhythm, the strengthening of social bonds and the investment of meaning – which allow us to speak of rhythm dance therapy.

Has enthusiasm entirely disappeared from our dances?

The enthusiastic state triggered by popular dance is not a trance. This implies a loss of consciousness (e.g. such as we might find in voodoo). The individual who finds him or herself in a state of enthusiasm still maintains a certain presence of mind, transported, while remaining fully aware (e.g. the 'Mediterranean' trance as discussed above).

As a form of trance it is collective: the shared rhythm connects the dancer to the group and permits, as Euripides used to say, a 'bringing of souls together'. Everyone celebrates the rhythm of life and exults in the feeling of being alive.

Rhythm also connects the dancer to himself by synchronising the registers which constitute the human being (i.e. physical, social, mental and psychic). The rhythmic repetition of movement causes a resonance between the organic and the psychic body: the body, the unconscious and the conscious self vibrate to the same rhythm, creating something new: another self. The energy pushes the dancer not only beyond the limits of the body, but also the limits of the ego. They reach the horizon of the unlimited which opens, becoming part of the stream of life which courses through the universe. The gesture, 'super-naturalised' by the rhythm, possesses the dancer the way the spirits and gods possess the patient in traditional therapies. They transform and heal through what anthropology calls *symbolic efficacy*.

In the West, despite a strong interest in popular dance, its deeper meaning – that linked to a sacred resonance – has disappeared. As a result, dance has lost the therapeutic function which it had for our ancestors and which they conserved in our traditional societies. Can today's dance therapy detach itself from the precious heritage of trance dance which disappeared in the West because religious, political and intellectual powers suppressed something which they considered to be savage and wild?

Popular European medieval dances were the victims of the universal repression of popular culture (demonised because they were linked to magical beliefs and pagan superstition). Yet, rather than inducing states of demonic trance, they were characterised by scenes of jubilation. This has provoked suspicion from religious authorities since Saint Augustine (Legendre, 1978). The movement to suppress dance grew in intensity from the Middle Ages, culminating in the bloody

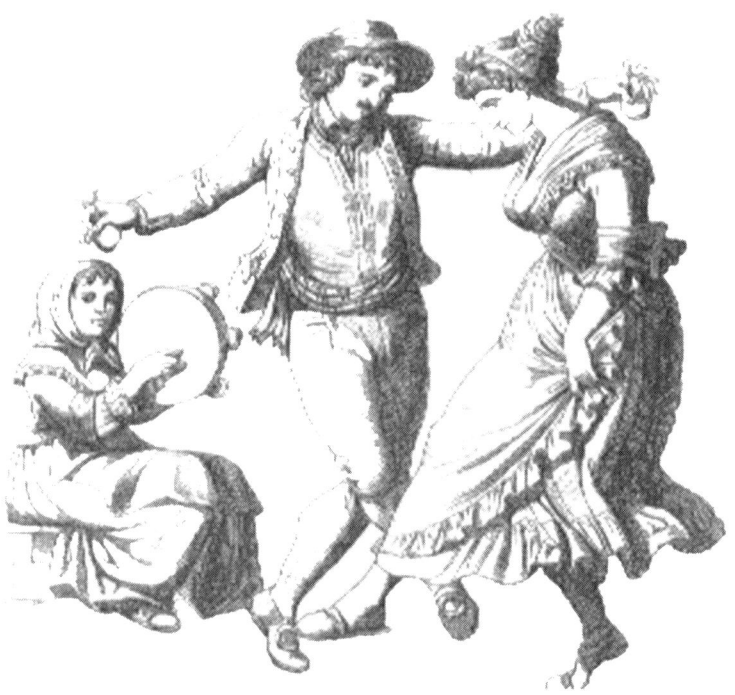

Figure 4.1 An example of a variety of courtship tarentella dances practiced today
Source: Drawing by G. Gambardella

repression of the *sabbats*, popular nocturnal assemblies where people danced and enjoyed festivities in the eighteenth century.

Our popular dances have been devalorised and marginalised, and therefore dispossessed, to a large extent, of the therapeutic power they once held within the socio-cultural context. Codified and classed today as folk dances, they are no longer invested with sufficient meaning to be in a position to support the therapeutic process of symbolic reorganisation.

This loss of our 'primitive' European heritage is not without its consequences. We see today, particularly amongst the young, the desire to re-create the rhythmic, pulsative, repetitive and collective forms of music (e.g. rock, techno or hip hop) inspired by jazz and tribal dances. Indeed for a number of commentators, this represents new rites in search of their myth (Le Breton, 1990: 13–28). Despite the loss of meaning which prevents the application of popular dances as a form of therapeutic intervention in a strict sense, their insistent rhythm still harbours powerful therapeutic potential. This can be seen in terms of their ability to create group cohesion and bonds between individuals. They awaken a sense of harmony and have the capacity to stir emotions and to release successive waves of pleasure through the rapid growth of their *tempi*. Their successful application in care centres is, therefore, not surprising.

Around the world, the triggering and harnessing of modified states of consciousness are at the heart of the traditional, therapeutic practices grouped together under the term 'shamanism'. These dances were suppressed within our societies, yet have returned with a vengeance today in the West. This revival, however, also harbours certain dangers. There are many who seek to harness the therapeutic potential of these dances without having studied their traditions, and who content themselves with the superficial use of randomly selected symbols as magic formulas bereft of any psycho-anthropological perspective.

Wary of such misapplication, we will now turn our attention to the healing technique of shamanism with a view to proposing a modern dance therapy capable of drawing on the work of countless generations of shamans, those ancestors of the art therapists of today.

5 Shamanism

Shamanism uses the states of trance to enter the supernatural world. The 'shamans' who still practise today across the world, from Siberia to Africa, from the Caribbean to Indonesia, are those individuals responsible for relieving suffering by acting as intermediaries between the invisible and human world. Contemporary shamanism has also developed urban forms, indicative both of its continuing vitality and openness to all human beings.

We will turn now to its teachings from a non-ideological perspective, exhibiting wariness towards the psychologising efforts of those involved in its contemporary appropriation, such as we find in New Age religion which is an appropriation of shamanism without real anthropological understanding. Such an appropriation subverts the spirit of shamanism to the objective of the quest for a narcissist self, which is far from the objectives of, for example, the Native American shamans, who search to apply the laws of the earth to humanity.

The search for the meaning of shamanism within the project of re-orienting dance therapy, through techniques which have proved their worth over millennia, will lead us to discover the coherence of a system with a structural unity that can be traced across the world. In a similar way to which anthropology has sought to draw a parallel between the work of the shaman and the psychoanalyst, I will seek to demonstrate the continuity between shamanism and dance therapy. I hope to pursue the work undertaken by contemporary anthropologists who, following Claude Lévi-Strauss, seek to explain the more disconcerting aspects of shamanism by demonstrating that the archaic rituals of the 'primitives' are not without their echoes in our modern world.

Universality and the persistence of shamanism

Archeological traces attest that shamanism was already present in the Paleolithic period. The *Trois Frères* cave in the Pyrenees contains a painting which is 15,000 years old in which we can see, at the centre of a group of gambolling animals, a dancing shaman, covered in lion skin, tracing an arc (Figure 3.2). Anthropologists surmise that shamanism was in existence even before this.

We are not dealing here with a religion, if we understand by religion an institutional system involving clergy and dogma. Shamanism corresponds rather to the underlying bedrock of religion, to its essence. It would, as such, be more accurate to definite it as a pre-religious phenomenon.

Shamanism emerges from the conviction of *Homo* that there is another order, a 'second world' – a hidden reality which suddenly flourished in the cultural productions of our most distant ancestors. *Homo sapiens* were, above all, shamanic humans in a dialogue with an invisible world, peopled with spirits communicating through the plants, trees, stones, animals and stars. One ethnologist who in a state of irritation exclaimed reproachfully to a Balinese shaman 'But where do you see those gods of which you speak? I don't see them anywhere!' received the reply of the surprised shaman: 'But where do you not see them?'

In shamanism, the link between nature and the spirits is assured above all by the shaman, the mediator between two worlds, through his ecstatic experience. According to Mircea Eliade, ecstasy, the state of 'leaving the self', is structural to the human condition (Eliade, 1964). It is indeed practised by all primitive humanity, primitive man being, above all, an ecstatic being. Shamanism is 'among the archaic techniques of ecstasy' (Eliade, 1964), but we could refer instead to the more scientific notion of a 'modified state of consciousness', which equally designates a state of being transported outside of self. To settle the debate, the anthropologist Bertrand Hell proposed the term 'transitor' (*transiteur*). This illustrates the mediating aspect of the shaman who knows how to reach and give access to the second world (Hell and Collot, 2011: 60).

During my experience organising training sessions in Greece, I observed that the word ecstasy, in its fundamental sense of transportation outside of self, is currently employed there without religious connotation. It is in this sense similar to the word enthusiasm, which refers to a state of religious possession (to have a god dwelling within the self), yet which we habitually employ to describe everyday states of mind.

Although the term 'shaman' comes from Siberia, shamanism can be found around the world. According to the understanding of contemporary ethnology,

> 'the term "shaman" spread from the *Tungus* tribe where it originated to wider Siberia, then to North and South America, to Africa, India, China and South East Asia to designate the sorcerer-healer of the societies of oral tradition, reputedly capable of entering into contact with spirits or of being possessed while in a trance-like state'.
>
> (Mitrani, 1992: 133)

Although targeted by authorities, institutional churches, totalitarian regimes and the spread of science, shamanism remains a vital force in its traditional form and has indeed developed under new guises within the rational citadels of the West.

The diversity of its manifestations should not obscure the core meaning of shamanism: it is more than a religion. It explores and seeks to express the primordial and ecstatic relation of the human individual to the exteriority which permeates him, and thus manifests a deep knowledge of the human soul which remains relevant today.

For the shamanic system, nature is sacred, supernatural. Man is a component element of this sacred nature. One of the founders of modern anthropology, Lucien Lévy-Bruhl, saw the essence of the primitive soul in the feeling of participation (Lévy-Bruhl, 1922). Ecstatic trance is an experience of this link to nature which is at the same time 'super nature'. The tales of contemporary shamans attest to the permanence of such experiences: 'from Lapland to Patagonia, from the Paleolithic to the present day . . . the shamanic ordeals and the exaltation which follows in their wake are strangely similar (Halifax, 1991: 6).

The impulse to connect with our most fundamental roots attracts us today towards the shamanic system. In bringing to light its general interest for the human being, particularly in our era of loss of orientation, we will not follow the deconstructionist path which insists on the particular character of the shamanism of each region of the world. Rather we will take the trans-cultural path which searches for common traits: the trance and the shaman as healer.

An invisible world

Shamanism opens onto two worlds: the invisible and visible, which are profoundly linked in a continuous exchange which renders the entire universe living and coherent. It organises the circulation between the two kingdoms, permitting the human being to be a partner of an 'other' world: that of the invisible spirits which manifest themselves in nature. Ecstatic trance 'opens' the door to the supernatural permitting access to this 'other' reality. The shaman is a specialist in its application. Aided by his drum, and also sometimes by drugs, he voyages towards the spirits, speaking to them and searching them out in their world while conserving his mastery of self, his consciousness, control and memory, since he must recount, on his return, the events of his adventure. He may perform his narrative while immobile or while dancing and singing.

The shamanic voyage is a flight (Clottes and Lewis-Williams, 1996: 26)[1] which the shaman accomplishes often in the form of a bird, a universal symbol already present in Paleolithic shamanism: we see a shaman in trance in one of the frescos of the Lascaux caves, carrying a staff with a bird perched on top. This symbol can also be found in the shamanism of ancient Greece (Daraki, 1989: 187) and remains a constant of contemporary shamanism. In the 'magical flight' of the trance, the shaman voyages to the worlds of 'Above' and 'Below' to meet the spirits, demons and ancestors.

The theme of the descent to the underworld, the encounter with death, the dismembering of the body, the confrontation with demonic powers, the double nature, the circulation between death and life, the communion with the animal world found in both Dionysian and then Orphic mythology clearly shows the shamanic origin of Greek spirituality (Daraki, 1989: 187). Dionysius, half-man, half-god (or Orpheus who is closely related) or indeed the numerous Mediterranean gods who die violent deaths only to re-emerge from the underworld (e.g. Osiris, Adonis and Attis) all in some way attached to the bull are shamans.[2] The suffering which the shaman endures brings the world of play, art and festivity into being, in the same way that the murder of Dionysius by the Titans enables him to create rites of trance and of drunkenness of all kinds: not just of wine but of love, poetry and all the arts.

The shamanism which nourished the mystery cults, in which the essence of the spirituality of the ancient Mediterranean is expressed, may not perhaps have disappeared with their suppression at the hands of Emperor Theodosius during the fifth century AD. Might we not think of Christianity itself, with the sacrifice of Jesus on the cross, as a universal symbol of the reunion of opposites through the mutilation of his body (the side pierced by a lance, the forehead torn by a crown of thorns), his descent to Hell and his resurrection?

Shamanism is for all time and all cultures.

The shaman

It is because he is a master of the ecstatic voyage that the shaman is also a healer. This should not detract from the fact that the other participants are also led towards a state of modified consciousness via recourse to a diversity of techniques: through active participation in the animated, suspenseful retelling of his adventures; through the spectacle of the dance with its repetitive, hypnotic structures; through games, the conviviality of the banquet and even laughter. All these practices, considered today as mere forms of leisure, are 'obligatory' in the numerous shamanic rituals and contribute to their efficacy to such an extent that sadness and loss are frowned upon and regarded as responsible for their failure.

Trance involves setting up an exchange between two worlds, permitting the channelling of certain forces, of benefit to humans, from the invisible world. The worlds are made to echo each other through a play of homologies whose resonance induces the state of trance. The latter, therefore, harbours a cohesive potential, and can unify the human being by binding together the biological, social and psychological in a balance which must be maintained for health to be preserved. Such is the definition of the World Health Organization, which insists in corollary fashion that isolating these levels inversely constitutes a source of disequilibrium, therefore of illness.

The shaman is the master of the trance. He induces and masters his own state of trance while also inducing it in others. He possesses the tools which allow him to open the gates to the supernatural: drums, dance, masks, chants and mythical tales. Let us first meet this strange and fascinating person on whom so much ink has been spilt.

His image in the West has undergone a considerable transformation. From being viewed as a crazy magician-healer (Devereux, 1970: 14–31), the shaman is now more generally considered to be a therapist who accomplishes the transition from disorder to order, re-establishing harmony with both nature and culture. The question whether the shaman is either a 'disturbed individual', a neurotic, epileptic, psychotic, etc., or well balanced and intentioned, has long been the subject of controversy among ethno-psychiatrists. On the basis of much documentary evidence, Georges Devereux, an advocate of the psychopathological interpretation and current ethnology, sees this figure more often as an individual who has indeed known the disorder of illness and its personal difficulties, yet who has surmounted them and emerged stronger, acquiring along the way the capacity to help others. As Mircea Eliade puts it, the shaman is not merely a sick man but rather a sick man who has succeeded in healing himself.

The shaman is a charismatic individual, possessing supernatural powers and, as such, is capable of establishing relationships with invisible powers, visiting their kingdoms and serving as an intermediary between man and the world of spirits. He uses magic and the supernatural to become a mediator between the forces of nature with which he speaks in the 'language of the spirits' and the human community to whom he speaks the language of his culture. The bird-shaman ascends to the skies and performs all kinds of metamorphoses thanks to the aid of his auxiliary spirits, animals, plants, or rocks. He represents the fulcrum for the continuous exchange between nature and culture, poised on the threshold of the gods. He flies towards the Heights and Depths, assisted by a bear, dog, eagle, stag, horse or plumed serpent. Both artist and performer, he describes his ecstatic adventure through song and dance, but also employs theatre, masks, mime, poetry and mythology.

Not everyone can become a shaman. He must experience a supernatural election communicated through a series of messages (dreams, visions, 'wild' trances, or illness (Schott-Billmann, 1985: 39–44)). His progress must be watched over by another shaman. He must pass through difficult ordeals (e.g. fasting or isolation), carry out an apprenticeship in techniques and esoteric knowledge, and memorise chants and dances. The future shaman must also possess artistic talent and be capable of improvising, placing his personal stamp on a heritage passed down from previous generations.

The shaman has paid the price for being able to cross the boundary between the supernatural and human world. He has descended to the underworld, his body dismembered by the infernal spirits. He has encountered death and defeated it by making the demons his allies. As we observed, every shaman has undergone painful ordeals (death, separation, illness, for example, as a child) and the idea of mortal suffering is an essential element in the election.

His stay in the country of the dead has given the shaman knowledge of the opposites: death and life, the world of the visible and invisible, presence and absence, life and death, and so on. He has reconciled the opposites within himself and, as such, possesses a double nature, both human and non-human. His clothes of animal skin are a sign of his connection to the animal-supernatural world. For the shaman, a true Spinozist, the divine is one with the natural.

Once initiated, the shaman does not 'rest on his laurels'. He must show that he is capable of meeting the needs of the members of his community: taking care of the sick, giving advice, organising rituals, etc. He is an authority in many areas: priest, sage, diviner, doctor, teacher, all-round artist (musician, singer, dancer, storyteller, poet) and a guardian of folklore. We should also remember that the term 'shaman' can be masculine or feminine – women are also called to this vocation.

The practical efficacy of the work of the shaman is now accepted by anthropologists. The position of Nadel (1949), cited by Lévi-Strauss, illustrates such belated recognition: 'under the influence of contact with civilization, indeed it seems that the frequency of psychoses and neuroses tend to rise, in non-shamanic groups, under the influence of contact with civilization, whereas in shamanistic groups it is the shamanism itself which increases, but without any increase in mental disturbances' (Lévi-Strauss, 1987: 21).

Therapeutic tools

The shaman does not use his gift for his own personal gain. He maintains, moreover, an attitude of humility; he knows that the power he harnesses does not belong to him, but is merely 'on loan' from the supernatural forces of the universe. His election constrains him to put his skills to the service of the community and to fulfil his mission of maintaining equilibrium between the supernatural and human worlds.

The primitive societies of the hunter–gatherers already appealed to the services of the shamans, using magical rituals to ensure success in their search for food. Their services diversified with the advent of agriculture: mastery of the rain, prevention of disease and healing became the principal goals of those who had the ability to enter into contact with the sacred world and translate its ineffable language into ritual gesture.

Disequilibrium is expressed in the group in terms of sickness, a bad hunt, a disastrous harvest or an accident, and it falls upon the shaman to attempt to address the disorder, which translates into the search for a lost soul, a frequent etiology of sickness in the shamanic system. To phrase it in contemporary terms, the shamans have always attached much importance to the psychic roots of illness, and as such their technique resonates with a modern medicine ever more aware that sickness is often the message our body sends to us to warn us of something.

The shaman, envisaging illness as a loss of soul, embarks on his search to regain it by using the 'ecstatic' voyage to fulfil his mission. His 'weapons' are the drum, incantation, dances, chants and symbols which permit him to translate illness and the process of healing into mythical narrative. We will now examine these one by one.

Drum

The use of the drum is universal in shamanism. It is the preferred instrument of the shaman and its obsessive, monotone character helps him to embark on his voyage. Hallucinogenic drugs are used in certain cases, but the drum alone is a powerful means of inducing a trance and has the advantage of avoiding secondary effects. In anthropology, the importance of the drum is often underestimated. Perhaps it is too self-evident, yet does not the reminder of the beating of the maternal heart in the rhythm of the drum provoke a return to archaic depths, to a primordial lived experience?

Song and chant

Singing and chanting are the vehicles of the spirits, expressed in a melodic and rhythmic fashion through the voice of the shaman. For each spirit there corresponds a specific form of song or chant recognised by all participants. This allows them to identify the power which manifests itself or is invoked by the shaman.

Siberia is a good starting point for an analysis of these chants (Helimski and Kosterkina, 1992: 37–51). For the Siberian tribe of the Nganasan, metre and poetry constitute the discourse of the spirits. Poetic metre serves to render discourse sacred, allowing it to be addressed to supernatural powers or to their emanations. The goal of the incantation is to distance harmful powers and to attract the attention of the spirits to engage in dialogue with them. A typical model involves eight syllables with the accent on odd syllables and a caesura after the fourth. Octosyllables make up 90 per cent of chants, while the remaining 10 per cent are devoted to improvisation which within this tribe is the responsibility of the shaman who adds a spontaneous segment to stereotyped formulas. In other societies, the Salish Indians of North America, for example, participants are also given an allotted time in which they can improvise during the 'dance of the spirits'. Singing in both a ritualised and rhythmic fashion, in interaction with the group, can be as cathartic as crying.

It would be interesting to study in greater depth the special bond between rhythm and the presence of the sacred and to clarify the relation between coded chant and improvised chant. What also remains to be carried out is an analysis of its different mode of expression from the varying perspectives of individual, collective (in terms of the unison of polyphony, canon, *ostinato*, etc.) and responsorial (the dialogue between the 'collective' and a 'soloist' shaman or participant). This would enable us to gain a better grasp of the structures most frequently employed. Contrary to what one might imagine, ecstasy which is a union with the 'other' (an exterior object, a powerful, supernatural divinity, mythical character, group, ancestor, animal or other entity of nature) does not necessarily take place either in silence or in the immobility of solitude. It can also be noisy and dynamic and occur within the context of a group performance. It involves an experience of plenitude, the 'rapture' of the mystics. Far from being locked in 'stasis', it is often expressed through the metaphor of magical flight, in the disappearing from view, ascending and descending to access different places in the universe. The theme of flight is universal within shamanism. We find in it numerous descriptions in South America, India, China, Tibet where shamans frequently use their drum to launch themselves into the immensity of the azure.

Numerous shamans enter into trance, in a conscious and controlled fashion, with the aid of dance. This raises the question of the relationship between dance and trance. Why should it be surprising that dance should illustrate this flight towards the sky or the underworld? Does not dance, above all, represent liberation from the weight of the self towards the heights or towards performance: a search for beauty, the absolute, a quest for transcendence? Dance can initiate such a voyage because of its particular capacity to harness the mimetic capacity of the human being to imitate not just the birds and other animals, but all the beings that he encounters and the events of his life. The shaman, who cultivates this capacity to a particularly high level, will use dance to express his adventures in the kingdom of the supernatural by miming the protagonists of the different episodes of this tale. Dance, poetry, chant and theatre are here inseparable. The dance of the shaman is a testament to the ability of this master of metamorphosis, during which he transmutes the savage forces of nature (present just as much within him as without) into a sacred, danced, theatrical performance, thereby channelling and containing them.

Dance

The shamanic dances are part of a wider group of tribal dances, also known as 'primitive' dance or, sometimes, 'ethnic dance' (this latter term refers also to 'folk' dance, whose primitive character has more or less disappeared). Their forms vary greatly between regions and cultures. As we have seen, they can be abstract, employing pure dynamics, or imitative: with the dancer, shaman or participant miming animal movements, social roles, trades, persons, etc.

Everyone must dance during the shamanic ritual in which the shaman is the master of ceremonies. He, therefore, casts an eye over the participation of each individual, by energetically banging his drum, reanimating the tired dancers, inciting the crowd to clap their hands and sing to accompany the collective dance. They must be in trance![3] The shamanic dances of the group often take place within the framework of rituals which prepare for war, imitating bellicose attitudes and gestures, or hunting rituals which involve the imitation of animals with a view to appropriating their qualities in order to hunt them better. During the dance of the spirits of the Salish Indians of the Pacific East Coast of North America,

> 'The spirit of the dancer finds its theatrical expression through step, rhythm, movements, postures and gestures: through the furtive step, then bounding leap of the warrior who lets out ferocious cries; through the slow tread of the big mother bear who moans sadly and cries for her missing cubs; through the father lizard who sheds tears over his devoured child, or through the imposing whale who catches the little fish. The choreographic drama of the dance of the spirits becomes thus a psychodrama associated with an emotional discharge of a cathartic type within the group.'
>
> (Jilek, 1992: 33)

Such dances are always carried out for life and for the living. The Dance of the Spirits, for example, was reinterpreted during the 1960s to symbolise the death of Indian culture, followed by its resurrection. There are shamanic dances which, while orientated towards resurrection, underline, above all, the theme of sacrifice. This is true of the celebrated Sun Dance of the Sioux, which was forbidden in 1881 only to reappear during the early 1960s. This is very much a therapeutic dance, directed by a shaman. To the rhythm of chants, drums and eagle bone whistles, the dancers, whose skin is pierced by hooks attached to a central pole, move progressively further from this pole while dancing around it. They do this four times, by which time their body is lacerated, incarnating the theme of the dismembered body universal within the shamanic tradition. Through its mortifying character, this dance illustrates the necessity of visiting both worlds, the world of the dead as well as the living, to establish an exchange between them. The dancers become the membrane which vibrates between these worlds like the skin of the shamanic drum, linking thereby the opposites through rhythm and the renewal of life.

The theme of two opposed worlds is a constant in shamanic dance. It is played out in an exchange between binary pairs whose opposition is thereby exceeded through their repetition and in the vector of upward movement constitutive of magical flight. The union of death–life and visible–invisible is the objective of trance. Repetitive dances could be called 'Dionysian', even if they are not Greek (e.g. tribal African dances), insofar as, similar to the ancient mysteries, they are based on eternal return. As the movements reproduce themselves identically, it is as if the dancers are confronted with the infinite return of the identical. Time is, therefore, abolished for the subject himself who finds in repetition the assurance of always being alive. We should remind ourselves that shamanic dances aim to 'renew' life. In the movement through which action erases itself and returns, dies and is reborn, we glimpse an irrepressible force of life, a kind of permanent resurrection, a victory against death. Assured of the return of the anticipated event, the dancer can deliver himself to enthusiasm and the pleasure of anticipation. The effacing of the gesture announces its return; desire resurges continually from its disappearance like the phoenix reborn from the ashes.

Dance is thus addressed as a message to the unconscious of the dancer: the 'shamanic' secret of the victory of life over death. Yet we must not understand this in the Christian sense of resurrection after death. It concerns man in the present. In effect, the repeated movement not only returns in an identical fashion, but is each time more powerful. The desiring being, invested in the movement of growth through repetition, is thus called upon to exceed his or her limits. The philosophical content of primitive dance, which is driven by a kind of 'dynamic meditation', is to be understood both in relation to the species – each generation raises itself stronger than the one which proceeded it – and in relation to the individual for whom each day brings a renewal of energy and fresh hope in progress. Dance displays desiring man; it is, in its incarnated manifestation, epiphanic of the subject of desire that human immortality resides. If, as Nietzsche insists, the word 'Dionysian' expresses an exceeding of the horizon of the self, the shamanic dances, the primitive dances express the Dionysian essence of human existence which is celebrated in dance and expressed through its intoxication (Commengé, 1988: 209). Does not the dance share the exaltation of Zarathustra as he climbs ever higher, until the stars are below him?

The mechanism of regular repetition is conspicuous in the productions of 'primitive arts' (Boas, 2003: 14).

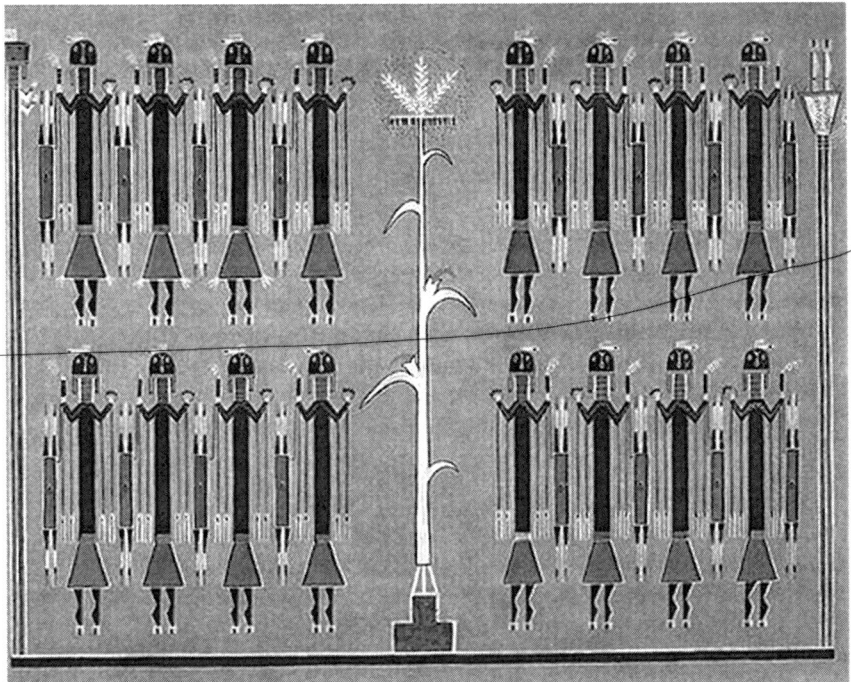

Figure 5.1 Navajo sand painting
Source: agcra.typepad.fr/navajos

The regular repetition animates the rhythm of primitive dances, which are characterised by an indefatigable re-launching of movement (Figure 5.1). The basis of their step, and often its only form, consists in an alternating of the feet to a regular beat and repetitive rhythm as the basis for the movements of the body which themselves are perpetually reinitiated. The dance of the *Anasterarides* in Greece, which is of pre-historical origin, is limited to a perpetual movement of the feet back and forth in front of icons (Schott-Billmann, 2006: 169–177). Other primitive dances systematise and generalise various movements of the body according to such repetitive dynamics. Repetition transforms those who perform them into 'champions' of a desire perpetually renewed, thereby into paradigms of human existence. It equally serves to strengthen the bond between dancer and the gesture inherited from his or her ancestors, each one becoming progressively more 'enamoured' of the other. As the source of its vitality, the encounter between the dancer and external gestural form serves to translate the encounter between the 'I' and the ideal 'Other' with which the 'I' must bond for it to function as the medium for its self-representation. The study of primitive dance, therefore, serves as the key to grasping the nature of dance as such.

All tribal dances and a considerable number of folk dances issuing from them are constructed on the basis of the repetition of movements. Their discourse is not linear but circular: the arrow of time is abolished since the event represented by the danced action is always reinitiated. Repetition is inseparable from rhythm, which re-launches the movement of the dancer with ever-greater intensity and dynamism. It pushes the dancer to exceed his or her own limits, towards a state of incandescence: a transportation 'outside of oneself'. Carried by successive waves, the gestures are performed with ever-greater ease – we might say that they 'perform themselves'. The dancer can take delight in them to the point of intoxication: he or she is progressively suffused with a movement which returns infinitely to the point of vertigo. By virtue of their rhythm and repetitive character, primitive dances always involve enthusiasm and trance. Emanating from the outside, from another who corresponds to an ideal (whether embodied by tradition, the shaman, the master, or another dancer who is more experienced), the gesture becomes the representation of this outside, of this ideal 'Other'. Through a circular movement uniting both two 'partners', gesture and dancer, when the dancer 'possesses' (masters) the gesture through its repetition, the latter 'possesses' the dancer and causes him to 'embark' on an exhilarating voyage. The dancer unwittingly transforms, indeed transfigures, the gesture by allowing it to display, through his own body, all its 'supernatural' beauty, the invisible beauty which we know as the presence or grace of the dancer.

While shamanic dance may, at times, appear far removed from dance therapy, at the heart of both is the same harnessing of repetition. By consolidating the bond between the movement and the one who performs it through its repeated performance, primitive dance designates the latter, with ever greater insistence, as the author of the performance. It heightens the dancer's feeling of acting, thereby sharpening their feeling of existing.

Mythological representations

To describe his adventures in the supernatural and invisible world, the shaman makes use of mythology and his creative imagination. This is different from the personal imagination: shamanism envisages human existence within a framework of cosmic symbolism. The universe is a personalised cosmos: a macrocosm. All its mysteries, such as the sun, the moon, the cycle of seasons and everything we encounter in nature, emanate from invisible powers. The human being is himself a microcosm reflecting this macrocosm like a mirror, desiring only to enter into phase with it in ecstasy: resonating with the plants, animals, other men, living and dead, the stones, rocks, waters, stars and the entire cosmos.

The powers of the universe have names. Amongst the Inuit or Eskimos, for example, the mythical original ancestors are Grandfather Fire, Grandmother Growth, Father Sun and Mother Earth. Certain animals have the status of less-distant ancestors, such as Bear, or symbolise powers of the Earth, such as Serpent. Elements such as the Sun or Mother Earth are also found in archaic Greek religion and can still be seen at work today in the traditional carnivals of the

Mediterranean. In Sardinia a dance of masked man-bears (the *Mammotones*) carry out acrobatic leaps while ringing bells attached to their fur.

In Northern Greece, we still find the dance called *Kaloyero,* the 'good old' one. This 'carnival man', a Dionysian character clothed in animal skin, is also covered in bells, and possesses a mirror whose function is to ward off evil spirits. On numerous Greek islands, 'animalised' characters wearing fur, masks and bells, perform primitive dances based on leaping and turning, contrasting sharply with the subtlety of Greek folk dances. We should note that vestiges of this ancient Dionysian shamanic practice can be recognised in several European carnivals (e.g. in Binche, Belgium, and in Basle, Switzerland).

Other important symbolic objects are the rainbow, the 'bridge' to the other world, and the crystal, the 'seed' of rebirth. The latter is employed today in somewhat distorted fashion by the neo-shaman when he advises his patient to place beside himself a 'crystal' orientated towards the sun to receive beneficial energy. It is dangerous to use the highly symbolic system of the shaman under the guise of a 'recipe' to be taken literally without embedding it within its cultural matrix (except here a vague concept of 'energy' which, from the sun, would pass through the crystal, then into the body) and without a transposition, which the anthropological study of its mechanisms would alone render possible. We do not easily enter into contact with the 'supernatural' (the invisible or unconscious). It requires the harmony of a symbolic resonance which creates ecstasy through ritualised practices refined over a long period of time.

Dance can serve as an example of such a practice: if it involves a musician who is truly at the service of the group and if it serves to put to one side the expression of 'me and my emotions', the dancing body participates in the body of the universe. Viewing shamanism from the perspective of dance would contribute thus to the renewal of the shamanic heritage while giving the body its rightful place within it. It would also avoid the distortions of certain contemporary movements of the 'New Age' which are not sufficiently anthropological in their understanding of this heritage.

The shamanic cure

The shaman is a healer and our societies still retain, at their margins, certain practices of shamanic origin: healers of various types and hypnotists, among whom there are certain who practise magic in a more-or-less veiled fashion, using the powers of particular plants (the mandrake), animal substances (milk of the female ass, sperm of the toad), stones (jasper, since it is red and thought to stop haemorrhages) or rhymed formulas (the fire healer burns while reciting secret phrases). At first glance, the perspectives of shamanism and those of western biomedical discourse appear irreconcilable. Shamanism see the world as a living and coherent whole, whereas medical and scientific culture analyses, classifies and names objects perceived in the world or our body by treating them as discrete 'entities'. Yet it is precisely the intercommunication of all elements of the universe, the vision of a continuous fabric linking men, animals, plants, rocks and even stars, which is without doubt an important factor behind the contemporary interest in shamanism. Would it be ill-advised to seek to unite two visions of healing beginning from such fundamentally different hypotheses? On the one hand, there is shamanism in which all is linked, including the present and the past, with its '*homo shamanicus*' meeting with the wind, sky and rivers, sharing their secrets and stories. On the other hand, there is science in which all is separated, with its '*homo scientificus*' firmly rooted in the objective world, who cannot accept psychic phenomena as real facts and who is scandalised by the current expansion of 'subjective sciences' such as astrology, the divinatory 'sciences', chiromancy and physiognomy. Yet, rather than oppose such sciences polemically to the exact sciences, it appears to us more fruitful to attempt to understand why these 'parasciences' today enjoy such renewed interest, however frustrating this might be for the scientific spirit orientated towards objectivity.

The attraction of our contemporaries to these disciplines is due, in large part, to the desire to play a role oneself in the healing process: not to be reduced to the role of passively absorbing medicines; rather to be active, stimulating our own mechanisms of self-healing. These aspirations are behind the present success of 'soft medicine' which proposes a personalisation of the healing process (such as we see when homeopathy adapts its molecular prescriptions to the 'field' of the patient) and a taking charge of oneself. It is not uncommon for a cancer patient to decide in conjunction with the practitioner of alternative medicine his or her regime of care and 'natural' ritualised actions, such as taking cold showers at fixed times of the day, physical exercise, and so on. In any case, what the study of the techniques of shamanic healing demonstrates is that they are not fundamentally at odds with modern medicine which, for its part, has also turned towards a personalisation of the cure and the activation of the processes of self-healing stimulated and supported by symbolic, ritualised activity (dieting and lifestyle management) among which we should include arts therapy and, in particular, rhythm dance therapy.

An example of shamanic healing

Thanks to anthropology, shamanic cures and their therapeutic mechanisms are now better understood. This should encourage therapists to follow Claude Lévi-Strauss' advice to psychoanalysts and measure their work against this millennia-old heritage (Lévi-Strauss, 1963: 204).[4] Dance therapists should pay particular attention, given the importance of dance in shamanic rituals. They can only benefit from an anthropological approach to the revitalising of such traditions, in which the goal is not merely to relive the past, but to create a therapeutic technique which takes inspiration from them, while remaining firmly rooted within the sensibility and knowledge of the twenty-first century.

Lévi-Strauss indicated such a route in his famous chapter (Lévi-Strauss, 1963: 186–204) whose analysis of the cure seeks out the foundation of the therapeutic mechanisms of shamanism. He attempts, namely, to understand the procedures of the Indian shaman from the tribe of the Cunas in Panama, called to heal a pregnant woman whose life was in danger. At no point did the shaman touch the body of the patient. Rather, he gave expression to her sufferings through an epic chant, translating her pain into the language of myth. This was all that was required to heal her. The myth is a kind of simulacrum, rooted in the mimetic instinct. As in theatre and dance, miming a model leads to a metamorphosis of the human body. For Lévi-Strauss, the key condition is that the myths proposed by the shaman must be 'lived intensely'. This intensity derives from the power of the bond which unites in a reversible exchange the individual and the object endowed with potency. It explains how the myth proposed by the shaman acted corporeally on women in labour: through the homology between the female reproductive pathways and the cave and corridors followed by the shaman and his auxiliary spirits before emerging into the open air. In the therapeutic practices of the traditional healer the use of simulacra 'calls' the forces of the cavern and subterranean passages to 'respond' in the body of the patient by acting on his own cavities and conduits to liberate the child.

Lévi-Strauss uses this example to pinpoint the essential therapeutic mechanism of the shamanic system: symbolic effectiveness. Citing Desoille, the inventor of guided imagery, he reminds us that 'psychopathologic trouble is only accessible to the language of symbols' (Lévi-Strauss, 1963: 199). Shamanic mythology offers a wide range of such symbols. When the myth proposed by the shaman is 'experienced intensively' by the patient, an ecstatic communication is established between the latter and the invisible world – a correspondence between the psychic and supernatural. The shaman mobilises mythical persona via a narrative which 'unblocks' the pathogenic situation. This is translated into a corresponding 'unblocking' acting at the level of the psyche and of the body of the sick person, one which, in this case, culminated in the birth of the woman's child. This mythical transposition allows the sickness to be transposed and to flow in cathartic fashion into symbolic forms.

The interest of this 'mythologisation' of the psychism has not escaped certain psychoanalysts. Jacques Lacan recognised the transposition of psychic characters into divinities as a procedure which works in a similar way to psychoanalysis. He expresses this in somewhat raw fashion: 'there were shovelfuls of gods – all one had to do was find the right one. Which led to this contingent thing that is such that sometimes, after an analysis, we manage to achieve a state in which a guy correctly fucks his "one gal"' (*sic*) (Lacan, 1998: 115).

The difficulty for us westerners derives from the fact that the gods, which the shamans perceived just as clearly as we do our houses or cars, have today deserted us. We will have to appeal to another symbolic system if we are to make use of the anthropological rereading of the shamanic cure and take inspiration from it.

The ambition of dance therapy is to harness the capacity of dance to link the self to the outside world and to the Other. We agree with the Indian shaman when he states that 'a good object of medicine links all the worlds'.

In the same chapter, Lévi-Strauss makes a comparison between psychoanalysis and shamanism, in which he asserts that both are based on a mechanism of symbolic effectiveness. They offer the drives a form of release through a language which articulates them through symbols, reorganising the psyche through words. Anthropology is thus in full agreement with psychoanalytical theory. Here, the cure consists not only in the discharging of repressed or conflicting drives, but also in linking them to new representations. Both methods accomplish this in their own fashion: shamanism through the symbols of supernatural powers; psychoanalysis through words symbolising psychic lived experience.

Lévi-Strauss identifies another difference between the two types of cure. While the psychoanalyst listens to the patient, the shaman is the orator and speaks for him. The first acknowledges the words emitted by the individual lying on the couch; the second brings symbolic representations to the cure from outside. We may say that the shaman 'injects' into his patient a symbolic language drawn from an already available set of collective representations. The sick person listens to the mythical encounters and internalises its symbolic form in a centripetal movement. These forms engage with his illness, awakening and addressing it directly to channel and express its effects. The success of their appropriation by the patient succeeds, the more he feels represented by them – the more he can funnel his drives, emotions, fantasies, memories through them. We find here the same centripetal movement as in the shamanic dances. The symbolic and collective forms, inherited from tradition and selected for their efficacy are offered to the participants through ritual: a channel through which their drive energies can flow.

Meaning and significance

Whether the myth is, formulated by the individual on the couch, or collective, received from tradition as in shamanism, the healing process corresponds to a reorganisation which is the work of the symbol.

The words employed by the shaman to describe the tale of the soul of his patient are carriers of a meaning which is not of the realist but mythical order. According to Lévi-Strauss, they would lose their effectiveness if they accounted for the pathological manifestation in mundane terms. The success of the cure demands the poetic 'travestying' of mythology (Lévi-Strauss, 1963: 197).[5] The anthropologist, indeed, suggests that truth is less therapeutic than symbol. Why is it that a description of viruses or microbes cannot cure flu, any more than the 'rational' explanation of parental misdeeds brings the neurotic out of his suffering, while a pure fabrication, a tale of monsters, for example, can heal a sick person? Lévi-Strauss risks a response, almost excusing himself for its paradoxical character: 'the reason lies in the fact that microbes exist and monsters do not' (Lévi-Strauss, 1963: 197).

This leads us to establish a distinction between 'meaning' and 'signification'. The first inscribes itself in forms which 'speak' to us and can represent us. The second corresponds more to the 'rational' unmasking of the psychic mechanism and of the causes said to be at the origin of the symptoms.

Art therapy is, in a similar fashion to shamanism, based on a 'veiling' of the truth under artistic forms, in an 'abandoning' of the illusion of the search for signification as the 'royal road of therapy' (Darrault-Harris and Klein, 1993: 54). Not all explanation heals: a heightened awareness of one's problem does not necessarily lead to a transformation of the person. Anthropology, in showing the value of the 'detour' of symbolisation, offers a valuable object of reflection to those therapeutic circles overly attached to a rationalising and prolix discourse which, by identifying the 'causes' of the illness, ultimately furthers the cause of the resistances to change. We know better today how much the desperate search for significance works against those who see in it the objective of psychoanalysis. Ever more 'conscious' and 'intelligent' in unearthing the motivating factors behind the psychic trouble (which is often only the illusion of knowledge), it ultimately remains tied to their symptoms, however much it knows 'why' these appear. As André Breton put it, 'lucidity is the great enemy of revelation'.

We should not conclude, therefore, that art therapy should promote obscurantism. Seeking above all the activation of the process of change in the subject through the 'meaning' invested in his artistic productions, the art therapist discovers one of the secrets of the shaman: it is through creating an 'another world' that the human can, if not decode, at least express its enigmas through artistic fiction, which is to say otherwise than in saying 'I'. The 'I' can thus say (itself) without the need to lay everything bare in the act of saying. If the healer appeals to symbol and simulacra, let us take care not to block, through an overly controlled 'secondary' and 'sober' discourse, the sick person's capacity to improve. Is not a good therapist, whether shaman or psychoanalyst, one who knows how to use play, as the 'Plays' of Winnicott and the '*Witz*' (play on words) of Freud and Lacan remind us?

The efficacy of symbolic acts

Lévi-Strauss indicates another promising route for art therapy, by reminding us that the symbol is not just a word, but also a rite, prayer and gesture. If psychopathological trouble can only be addressed through the language of symbols, verbal metaphors in the example in question, it is all the more accessible through symbolic acts. In effect, discourse, however symbolic, still comes up against the barrier of the conscious mind: we can 'reach deeply buried complexes only through acts', the 'concrete actions, that is, genuine rites which penetrate the screen of consciousness to carry their message directly to the unconscious' (Lévi-Strauss, 1963: 200). Referring to the work of a Swiss psychiatrist, the anthropologist adds: 'The gestures of Sechehaye reverberate in the unconscious mind of the schizophrenic just as the representations evoked by the shaman bring about a modification in the organic functions of the woman in childbirth. Labor is impeded at the beginning of the song, the delivery takes place at the end' (Lévi-Strauss, 1963: 200).

We should remember here that, while appearing to the West merely as a form of artistic expression, symbolic gestures are employed in traditional therapies within the framework of operations with precise objectives. Indeed, this component often plays a decidedly more important role in the operation of the shamanic cure than Lévi-Strauss's example of the woman in labour. Among the Araucan Indians, for example, mythical combat against harmful spirits is rendered theatrical. Among the Navajos, the sick person is successively placed in different localities in a gesture evocative of the composition of a giant painting. Shamans make use almost universally of masks to manifest supernatural powers in action.

We can draw two principal types of symbolic effectiveness from the anthropology of shamanic therapies: the first verbal, functioning via words; the second non-verbal, functioning via symbolic actions and closely related to art.

Let us add, finally, that traditional therapeutic systems are still regularly employed in numerous countries. The efficacy of its experienced practitioners, moreover, is now widely recognised not only by ethnologists but also by numerous psychiatrists open to the dimension of ethno-psychiatry; that branch of psychiatry which takes inspiration from these traditions in order to treat immigrant populations.

The therapeutic efficacy of rhythmic practices

The non-verbal forms employed by the Indian Cuna shaman, include gestures, music, rhythm and chanting voices. The myth proposed to the patient is not pure text, since the words which constitute it take the form of a rhythmic chant. Moreover, the shaman recounts the myth whilst employing adapted obsessive techniques conducted at a frenetic pace. This leads us to raise the question of the therapeutic role of rhythm, music and dance in shamanic cures. Lévi-Strauss did not venture into this domain. Yet their almost universal use in traditional cures suggests that art is used systematically in shamanic therapies, the ancestors of the art therapy of today, which leads us to the following question: do musical and gestural symbols constitute incidental supports of mythical speech or do they harbour their own therapeutic potency?

The example on which Lévi-Strauss bases his analysis involves incantation, rhythmic and repetitive chants, in which the shaman transposes the drama of the parturient into a narrative of the quest for the lost soul. We will attempt, however, to abstract from the layer of explicit meaning to bring out the therapeutic function of the chanted voice, melody and rhythm, thereby supplementing the Lévi-Straussian analysis of the symbolic effectiveness of the words of myth with an analysis of the artistic forms which support it.

Reactivation of the archaic relation to the mother

The role of the shaman who sings evokes the mother vocalising for and with her child: cradling it, proposing all sorts of games of the voice and body. If art therapy can take inspiration from the practices of shamans, the latter seem to have been keen observers of the way in which all human mothers relate to their child through an ensemble of corporeal rhythmic and vocalised activities. If the mother–child exchange possesses both a pedagogical and therapeutic function, in the wider sense of the prevention of psychic troubles, it can legitimately be adapted to operate within the framework of curative therapies. Do these not reactivate ancient situations which, when experienced negatively, engender illness, and when relived by the patient under favourable circumstances procure the beneficial effects which failed to appear during their original enactment?

Psychotherapy is, in a certain way, an adapted pedagogy which allows us to draw on the traditional practices of both shaman and mother, activating through playful and non-verbal activities a structuring process accomplished above all through pleasure. In effect, the symbols harnessed by the shaman within rhythmic and vocal productions are active to the extent that they evoke the mother, functioning as 'maternal decoys'. There is, within these structures, an implicit dimension of commemoration and reactivation of situations which contributes to their emotional quality and increases their effectiveness.

Certain contemporary psychoanalysts, such as Dider Anzieu, are also adherents of this 'school' of the mother, searching out the different ways in which she offers the child first the pre-verbal, then the linguistic forms which facilitate the process of its constitution as a human subject (Anzieu, 1985).

When the mother carries out vocalisations and rhythmic games with her child, she offers to him, within this playful form, not only image contents but also structures. These are immediately recognisable in chants, poetic tales or dances: rhyme, association via assonant pairs (versification) and repetition (refrain), etc. In similar fashion to the mother in her relation to the child, the shaman who sings and chants offers the patient not only images, a lexicon and vocabulary for illness, but also structures defined by Lévi-Strauss as 'moulds which absorb the fluid multiplicity of the cases'. Let us clarify, however, that these structures are not arbitrary. To be effective, they must enable a commemoration reactivating archaic lived experience, thereby bringing it under a degree of control.

Arts therapy uses coded, structured and highly organised non-verbal forms (there can be no art without rules). Rhythm, chant and dance appeal to the deepest layers of the human, reactivating them and inducing the biological, psychological and social to resonate in phase. It is in this sense that we can understand the role of artistic forms which both connect and harmonise these different levels by virtue of their similarity to structures. This, in turn, allows for the transmission of beneficial modifications from one to the other in a positive reorientation which is at the heart of the therapeutic process.

Art therapy, in similar fashion to shamanic therapy, involves bringing the subject into contact with external structures through their homology to internal ones, thereby awakening, channelling, expressing and sublimating drives, emotions and fantasies. It proposes new representations which allow for a positive reorientation of the psyche, accomplished through joyful intensity and the full engagement of the body. Art therapy thereby represents a particularly effective technique for recreating the self by harnessing the power of symbols. Our study of shamanism raised one crucial question: can there be a therapy without the gods? After our overview of traditional therapeutic methods we may assert the validity of appealing, if not to divinities, then at least to symbolic representations which exceed everyday existence. Perhaps a certain degree of transcendence is always necessary for the individual when mobilising its humanity in its full intensity, in an 'exit from self' and a linking to objects which will enflame its passion and cause the self to resonate. Art is certainly the activity which enables most fully an escape from the ordinary and access to a 'second world' beyond the horizon of the self, a world centred on an ideal: the search for beauty.

This chapter has shown us that even if shamanism has elements in common with psychoanalysis, it finds itself in greatest proximity to arts therapy. Rhythm dance therapy occupies a privileged place within art therapy by virtue of its heightened capacity to put the body and the world into homological resonance. It is in equal measure capable, as we shall see, of accessing the traces left in the memory of the body by the phylogenesis (the history of the species) and ontogenesis (individual history) which lead us towards humanisation.

Notes

1 Shamans say they fly to faraway lands, or other worlds filled with spirits and monsters.
2 In commemoration of the sacrifice of Attis, the 'Gauls', devotees of the god, regularly castrated themselves in a state of trance, an act which was never tolerated by the official Roman religion.
3 Generally speaking, trance recuperates a lost force, drawn from 'elsewhere', and therefore plays a regenerative role, which explains why it is frequently at the heart of the rites of the renewal of life (of fertility, fecundity and the 'new year', etc).
4 '. . . psychoanalysis can draw confirmation of its validity, as well as hope of strengthening its theoretical foundations and understanding better the reasons for its effectiveness, by comparing its methods and goals with those of its precursors: shamans and sorcerers'.
5 'That the mythology of the shaman does not correspond to objective reality does not matter.'

Part III
The humanising process

6 The universe of fusion and its dangers

If ontogenesis recapitulates phylogenesis, the stages crossed by *Homo* to attain culture would be comparable to those of the child in following the path towards humanisation. Whether or not the analogy holds, an understanding of the path which each individual must follow in the course of their development is indispensable to the application of the cure. We shall start from the beginning, since no therapist who wishes to further their intuition through theoretically informed action can ignore the foundations of the human psyche and the fashion in which it is largely determined by the infant and its earliest relationships with those around it.

This knowledge is all the more necessary because dance therapy constitutes a privileged opportunity to reactivate its course. It serves to open a path towards regression to the archaic stages in the development of the self, along with its variants arising out of the lived experience of each individual, thereby offering participants access to their 'roots'. This allows us to reinforce the most fundamental levels of the psychic life of participants. It helps the latter to re-orientate and reconnect with these levels; to integrate within a renewed recognition of their self-identity.

The permeable body

For the sciences, it is evident that human existence participates in the universe. The human body is composed of the same atoms as stars and is formed from organic molecules identical to those found within all living creatures. It takes its place within the history of animal evolution which, from single-celled organisms, has, across time, evolved into our species. The human being is, therefore, in profound solidarity with the cosmos. Yet while primitive societies experience this feeling of participation in the world naturally through trance, our capacity for such experience has been significantly weakened by a series of ruptures disconnecting the individual from the world: the separation from the cosmos, the dualist division between body and mind, the individualist closure of the subject on itself, the forgetting of ancestors, and so on. The sentiment, rooted in the deepest levels of our experience, of being made of the same substance as the world, is not an easy notion for rational thought (as we understand it today) to digest. The animal participates unquestioningly in the harmony of the world. It 'is' the world; it 'is' the body. The human foetus, cradled in the womb and bathed in amniotic fluid, knows a state of continuity, of fusion, of non-differentiation with the environment, as does the newborn. This is a sentiment which Freud named 'oceanic' to underline the 'immensity' of the sensation of being a part of an 'All' in which no distinction can be made between self and the world, a sentiment which thereby draws us into infinity in an extreme dilation at work in diverse situations. Such experiences are sought after for the feeling of 'bursting' out of the self which they involve: states of drunkenness, not only via drugs or alcohol, but also through love, dance, poetry, music, language and the relation to divinity. Man has the ability to enter into 'fusion' with everything which exists. Trance, or ecstasy, could therefore be understood as belonging to the deepest layers of the self. Rhythm, in particular that of percussion, is crucial in inducing a state of ecstasy in that it reactivates the sensorial imprint of the stage in which the child hears the beating of the mother's heart. The drum also possesses an ability to lead the human being back to their primordial state. It, likewise, possesses the power to induce trance, which is why shamans the world over use it to this end. Trance is a product of the openness, or 'porosity', of the body which belongs not only to the subject, but is also permeated by the 'not-I', the 'Other': the forces of nature, the energy of the group, religious representations, and so on. This is why trance is a socially dangerous state, insofar as it induces the subject to transgress its usual physical and moral limits. Thus, we find in the primitive religion of Thrace, the Maenads who, in a trance state without any social limits, during which they are possessed by Dionysius, abandon their home, spouses and domestic tasks to go to the mountains and become true beasts of prey. They devour raw and still palpating animal flesh – even their own children (Euripides, *The Bacchanals*, 1912). However, even when trance is canalised, as in the dances, we have seen that in our society, it is subject to stigmatisation. It was attributed to the devil and repressed during the Middle Ages: such was the etiological explanation of the crisis of hysteria until Charcot and Freud. Yet, it has been conserved in numerous traditional societies in supervised and highly codified forms (e.g. the possession dances).

Have such experiences become so foreign to us? It is not necessary to be an ancient Greek or a member of an African tribe to feel exhilarated by contact with nature or a profound complicity with an animal: to feel oneself permeated, as Gilles Deleuze put it, by the 'becoming-grass' or 'becoming-tree'. Where do these states of trance come from?

Primary narcissism

In the world of fusion, the body is in osmosis with its environment; appears literally to absorb it. This 'porosity' of the exterior world probably has its origin in mimetism (see Chapter 2). The state of non-distinction between inside and outside, the 'fusion' between the world and the self corresponds in the human being to the psychic lived experience of the newborn where chaos reigns in a lack of differentiation between self and other, a state of 'adualism' (Piaget and Inhelder,

1984: 21). The psychoanalysts name this 'primary narcissism' in an allusion to Narcissus, who in Greek mythology lost himself in the contemplation of his own image. There is no 'other', all affectivity remains centred on self. Piaget, nevertheless, remarks that the use of the expression is debatable, for the good reason that where subject and object find themselves confused, there is no longer a subject. Without doubt, the expression 'symbiosis', proposed by Wallon, takes better account of this lack of differentiation in the very young infant who has not yet dissociated self and non-self, and who cannot thereby 'de-centre' himself.

Primary narcissism is a normal state for the newborn, not yet differentiated from the exterior world, and in particular from the mother who constitutes the first 'Other'. Lingering from the experience of the womb, primary narcissism is the sentiment of original existence. It is the foundation of an identity which constructs itself piece by piece. According to Françoise Dolto, it is via primary narcissism that we cultivate the feeling of having a body belonging to the human species (Dolto, 1984: 73). Primary narcissism provides us a first, very possibly genetic, representation of our humanity, with its own particular silhouette and face, even if representations of self linked to the experience of primary narcissism are very far from objective reality as the first drawings of children, albeit at a later stage of development, demonstrate.

The fusional state can also be dangerous and alienating. Because the body is in osmosis with its environment, it can literally absorb it by fascination, illusion and identification.

Fascination is a state of hypnosis which activates a mode of behaviour imperiously 'commanded' by the fascinating object. Fascination for one's self (like Narcissus) or for another is linked to the immobility of ecstasy. Humanity knows similar forms of fascination for vampires (or their incarnation as femme fatales or 'vamps'), mortal figures who fix their consenting victims to the spot. More generally, we feel the (fortunately) less dramatic fascination of love by allowing ourselves to be seduced by the presence in the other of traits which unleash a second type of hypnosis, a kind of possession.

Fascination represents a hypnotic mechanism inducing immobility, or a mimetic response, upon recognition of figures linked to predation (recognition of the 'hated' enemy or object) or to reproduction (identification of the object of 'love'). Fascination thus determines the 'choice' of object, a choice which is, in reality, largely passive. We remind ourselves that the decoy acts as a deceiving object with the capacity to confuse through the illusory image. Does not *homo sapiens* allow himself to fall into the same trap as the stickleback when he vibrates to the decoy of the object capable of inspiring hate or love for the one who bears it?

In reality, the human being allows himself to be fascinated and manipulated by lures all his life. He is entirely capable, without having faith in what they say, of following gurus for their beard wisdom, or leaders for their voice authority, to adore idols, defer to military stripes, lose one's head over a uniform or the opulence of a female cleavage, or indeed become sexually excited exclusively over curly hair, or brown or blonde, according to nature and the colour of the one who was the original prototype. The therapist, indeed, must be constantly wary of the danger that he or she might take on the aspect of a guru, or military chief or seducer, which is why we can never insist too much on the need for self-analysis.

The relation of the child to his mother is a clear example of fascination. An infant only reacts to her image when face to face. The mother, in profile, does not activate the child's smile, a response which is genetically programmed and induced by the lure 'eye-mouth'. We may indeed venture the hypothesis that the neurological immaturity which consigns the child to motor impotence produces an exceptional receptivity for fascination since it holds the child captive to the image, incapable of fleeing it. In particular, the image of the archaic mother engenders powerful impressions which are durable and sometimes very negative.

One patient, a pretty young girl, had imagined her mother to be a dangerous sorceress (an image inherited from the oral stage), and had constructed a subjective representation of herself, a body image which identified, despite herself, with this malefic figure. She perceived herself, just as much in her external aspect as in her 'devouring' relations to others, as a 'spider'. Although the identification in no way reflected her appearance, she could not perceive her own beauty, encountering in her reflection an ugly hag. To attempt to prove the opposite would have been a pointless exercise: her imaginary representation put a screen between her and the exterior world. Treatment consisted, therefore, of enabling her to free herself from this image inherited from the world of fusion and of proposing to her other non-pathogenic, autonomising forms of identification. The cure culminated in a magnificent dance of the spider performed by the young girl, inspired by the model of the Italian tarantellas, which, through its positive and valorising character, contributed to exorcising the sinister prototype that other cultures would have attributed to 'enchantment' or 'sorcery'.

We see here once again the fashion in which dance therapy proceeds by appealing to traditional pedagogical methods which have been employed for millennia. When a child is held captive by an anxiety-inducing image (fear of an unknown), or a disquieting fantasy (cries apparently without motivation), rhymed games and songs are used to help it escape. These facilitate liberation and de-fascination through the creation of substitute modes of behaviour (attack or flight), enabling the child to keep such troubles at bay. Later, when the child is capable, it appropriates these gestural and rhythmic forms to express himself.

Anthropology supplies numerous examples of the use of dance, song and rhythm to ward off 'malevolent images', evil spirits and dangerous powers. It would seem that the rhythmic hammering of the feet or clapping of the hands were sufficient to this end. Dance therapy equally makes use of such devices, where it is possible to neutralise pathogenic representations through the rhythmic play of the body and voice. This alleviates the anxiety of the participants as they are 'no longer thinking of anything'. Of course this represents only a partial harnessing of the therapeutic potential of such activity. It is no more than a temporary distancing of anxiety, a relaxation or 'clearing of the head'. We will see, however, that it also enables us to give to dangerous fantasies a language which neutralises their power to induce fascinating paralysis.

Illusion comes from our personal imagination which can influence our apprehension of reality to the point of deforming it. The psychotic is not the only human being to mix his fantasies (his interior world) with the exterior world. Man possesses an irrepressible tendency to confuse: not only the lure and the object in similar fashion to the animal, but also its fantasies and reality because the kingdom of the imagination is not limited to nocturnal dreams. *Homo sapiens* is forever recreating both the exterior and interior world through illusory doubles which make it 'think the moon is made of cheese'. The therapist has to pay attention to the fact that following the psycho-analyst Jacques Lacan, objectivity is impossible for us. We are constantly modifying reality, in particular through our relationships with others, interpreting them across the deforming prism of the imagination, endowing them with other qualities, faults, feelings, intentions largely fabricated by subjective vision. Psychoanalysis gives the name 'projection' to this defence mechanism which, for example, pacifies by absolving the self of guilt. We rid ourselves of this emotion by attributing to the other that which emanates from our own imagination, yet which cause us anxiety, hatred, or jealousy, etc. Even if the use of the imagination can be more or less controlled through the 'secondary process' of reason, the psychic life of the individual has to manage two realities: one concerns things, the other the mind in which he puts his faith. As Edgar Morin stresses, the advent of *homo sapiens* is also the birth of illusion, the reign of fantasy and hallucinatory satisfaction (Morin, 1973: 118–126). His relation with reality will, therefore, always be uncertain, full of error, subjectivity, chimeras, delirium and madness. If we add to this an emotiveness with a tendency towards convulsive manifestations (e.g. laughter or tears), an aptitude for paroxysmal states (e.g. ecstasy, drunkenness or orgasm) yet also suicidal depression, hatred or perverse *jouissance*, and if we consider finally that all these excesses, unknown in the animal, follow each other with such rapidity as to lead to incoherence, should we not follow the suggestion of Edgar Morin and re-baptise him *homo sapiens-demens*? We cannot hope to perform our duties as therapists correctly if we have not attempted to deconstruct our illusory personalities, neutralise their effects, and analyse their projections. It is only as such that we will be in a position to propose to patients a dance mediation which is not orientated towards our own ends and which does not transform them into so many screens for our own projections.

Body image

The propensity to imitate the other, to the point of assuming its physical appearance, is named 'identification' in psychology. The newborn corporeally 'absorbs' the emotions of his mother, which she transmits without her knowledge through her tone, posture, rhythm and the movements which he reproduces passively. Non-verbal elements vary and mark, in reflected form, the child's projected image of self.

Later, our identifications express themselves through our appearance – the way we dress, our hairstyle – indeed through our morphology. Some are beneficial, if their model is positive; they can also be pathogenic. Such is the case with archaic identifications to destructive figures which, against our will, we come to resemble. We have encountered several examples of these in dance therapy. One young man hated his father for his severe harshness, only subsequently to resemble him: identifying with the 'wolf', behaving like a ferocious animal, biting, 'howling' and even developing a *faciés prognathe*. Identification is comparable to the 'possession' of the body by an intruder. We are at first imprinted with the image of our parents in a passive way. We then 'ingest' their qualities through fantasy-driven oral incorporation before striving to resemble them to satisfy an ideal. We finally attempt to differentiate ourselves from them to find our own sense of identity.

Françoise Dolto, a famous child psychoanalyst, considers the postures and tonic variations interiorised by the child to be at the origin of the subjective representation of self-in-relation-to-the-others, an unconscious identity named in psychoanalysis the 'body image'. This is not only visual, as its name would suggest, but also synthesises the internal kinesthetic, postural, tonal and rhythmic sensations which constitute the imprint of the mother in her affective relationship with her child. The unconscious image of the body, initiated at the stage of primary narcissism, is modelled on the first moments of contact with the mother, in particular through contemplation of her face (the first mirror for the child, following Winnicott), her gaze and her different expressions. During the course of the development of the child, this image of the body undergoes a transformation measured by the progressive functioning of the diverse organs (e.g. oral, anal, phallic, genital). According to Paul Schilder, the body image 'is formed and structured by a perpetually renewed contact with the exterior world' (Schilder, 1968: 191). Dolto adds that it constitutes at each moment a living synthesis 'of our emotional experiences lived repetitively through the elective erogenous sensations, whether archaic or contemporary, of our body' (Dolto, 1984: 73). This image, in other words, can be modified according to the positive or negative character of the experiences and relationships we live through, because the game of mirror neurons continues throughout the life of the individual. We make full use of this possibility in dance therapy.

Dance therapy and body image

Body image, which is the result of successive identifications to people in affective relationships with the child, remains veiled and unconscious. Yet, as well as being apparent in the exterior appearance and body language of an individual, it can also be discerned in his fantastical productions: in dreams, and (of particular interest here) non-verbal creations. The latter involve not only human figurations of the body image, but also representations of objects, as well as animal life. Psychoanalysts often make use of sketching or modelling in certain moments of the cure or when the body image has difficulty migrating to speech, as is the case with numerous psychotics (Dolto, 1984: 73; Pankow, 1960). Unfortunately, these therapists often ignore dance and are thereby deprived of a precious means of accessing the body. In dance therapy, the body is the focus of attention. The careful eye of the dance therapist can detect in the dancer's movement traces of partial drives (oral, anal, phallic) and any defence mechanisms put in place by the subject. The, small, controlled, inhibited movements of the obsessive compelled by the anal drive of mastery and fearful of castration, who is therefore incapable of losing himself in movement, are a far cry from the expansive, animated and exuberant movements of certain hysterics strongly fixed to an orality which is both avid and generous. Professional dancers, however, do not represent good case studies for dance therapy as they can mask their body image by virtue of their mastery of the technique.

The dance therapist conveys to the dancer what he perceives of his or her image and invites the dancer to discover it after the session, confronting lived experience with observed spectacle. The video functions as a retrospective mirror and reveals much more than the mirror of the dance hall (forbidden because it hinders the 'letting go' necessary for trance): it unveils the body image. When confronted with the image of himself dancing, the participant is always surprised. The dance allows him to discover things about himself which he did not know. A slim young woman will discover that she dances as if her body weighs her down, thus becoming aware of the imaginary weight she attributes to her own body.

The fantasy of the dismembered body

There is no psychic unity at the beginning of human life; there reigns instead an incomprehensible chaos. The corporeal elements, far from being unified, appear scattered and diffuse to the infant, surging without warning from amidst the environment or floating in front of him. This strange perception of the world gives birth to a imaginary representation of the anatomy, leading to a body image which is anything but real. The parts of the body of his mother, confused with his own, call to the child and fascinate it as autonomous entities (Klein, 1950). This is particularly true of the breast, which interests the child to the highest degree, especially in the first months of its life. At the oral stage, all its activity, pleasure and relation with the surrounding world are centred on the mouth.

The different zones of the body which awaken successively during the course of development are underpinned by the experience of the physical functioning of the mouth (oral stage), the anus (anal stage) and the sexual organ (phallic stage). These partial drives are interwoven with others whose functioning implies the entire body (the drive for self-preservation, narcissistic drive, sexual drive, life drive, death drive), constituting a reservoir of drives called the 'Id'. In the child, they are not, at first unified, but dispersed and therefore dismembering. The 'fantasy of the dismembered body', has inspired numerous pictorial productions. It was vividly brought to life, for example, by Hieronymus Bosch, whose paintings abound in strewn body parts which are dismembered, dangerously autonomous and animated by persecutory intentions (Figure 6.1). The fantasy of the body cut into pieces is accompanied by anxieties of dismemberment, quartering, devouring, eventration, explosion, emptying of the body through the orifices, etc: terrible images which can always be observed at work among psychotics (who are

70 *The humanising process*

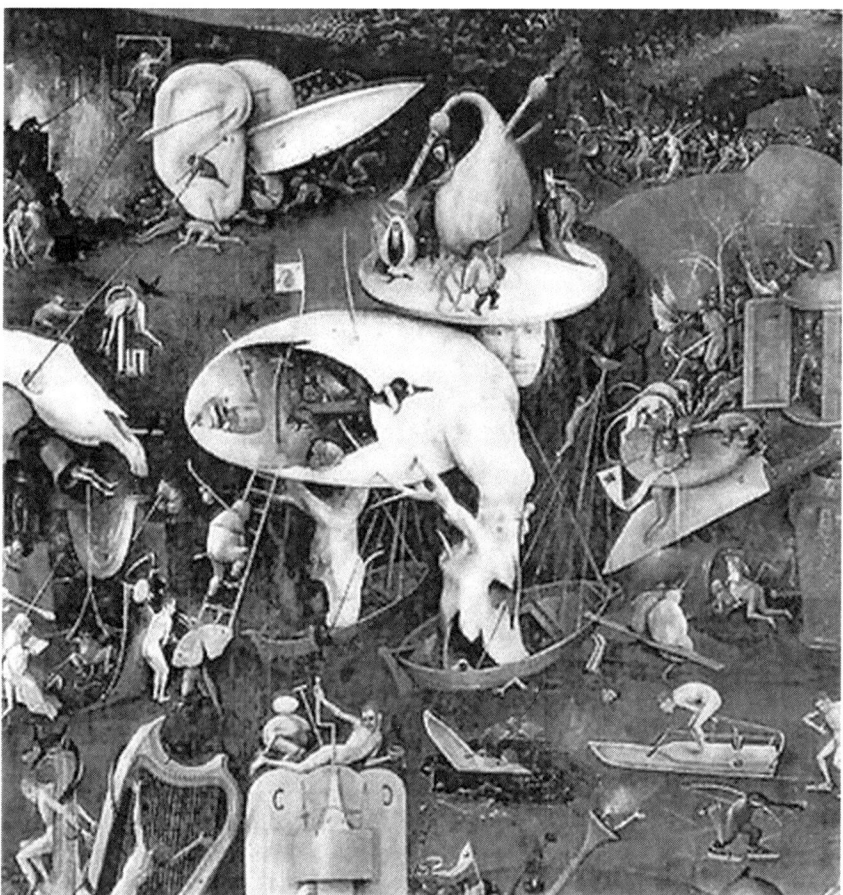

Figure 6.1 Detail of hell in *The Last Judgment* by Hieronymus Bosch, Academy of Fine Arts Vienna

subjected, thereby, to terrifying anxieties). It is the origin of the nightmares of children and of many phantasmagorical creations of tales and mythology: ogres, wolfs, werewolves, vampires and so on.

The renowned child psychoanalyst Melanie Klein worked extensively on archaic fantasies (Klein, 1975: 142). The drive objects split apart: the 'good breast', maternal, warm and protective, exists side-by-side with the 'bad breast', signalling absence and death. The child oscillates between these two imaginary perceptions of the mother tied to two poles: one positive and the other negative, linked respectively to the states of satisfaction or frustration. The first is associated with the image of the 'good breast' or the 'good mother' and the sentiment of 'love' for a beneficent figure; the second to 'hatred' for a destructive object. The 'bad breast' or 'bad mother' attacks and persecutes the child by means of a particularly terrifying object: the mouth, experienced as a giant abyss and perceived as an instrument of persecution which bites or swallows.

> I found that the aggressive impulses and phantasies directed against the mother arising in the earliest relation to the mother's breast, such as sucking the breast dry or scooping it out, soon lead to further phantasies of entering into her, the mother, and robbing her of the contents of her body . . . In such phantasies, products of the body and parts of the self are felt to have been split or separated from each other, projected into the mother and to be continuing their existence within her.
>
> (Klein, 1975: 142)

In mythology, the 'two mothers' are represented as good and bad fairies. We also find in these tales the seven key fears of young children linked to this primitive fantasy: dying of starvation, being devoured, poisoned, strangled, cut into pieces, emptied of substance or castrated. The pathogenic effects of the 'bad mother' are clearly at work in the negative body image, as we saw in the example of the 'young spider girl' above.

Persecution and fantastic retaliations risk 'exploding' the self. We see, therefore, the necessity, for the mother, of unifying the drives: containing them and integrating them within a holistic and positive expression. If this task has not been accomplished in childhood, it must be taken up by the therapist in the treatment of psychosis. To unify the dismembered body acutely persistent among psychotics, dance-rhythm therapy has, at its disposal, a particularly effective tool: rhythm, which synchronises the different parts of the body by making them beat to the same tempo.

Psychosis

Psychosis is a mental illness formerly known as 'narcissistic neurosis', a term which highlights its etiology. It is a result of the persistence of the initial state of fusion: with the environment and in particular with the mother. If all human beings conserve within themselves a 'psychotic core' inherited from their archaic past and nourishing certain fantasies, the pathology of the psychotic is the product of a psychic fixation at the 'symbiotic' stage. Carers will often say that the psychotic 'sticks' to them. Yet he can also be a prisoner of an imagination which he believes to reflect reality because it appears to him under the form of a (schizophrenic) hallucination, or see menace in everything, behave in a distant, hostile, furtive manner because he projects (psychotically) onto the people around him destructive intentions and feelings concerning his person, or because he fears his own drives which are dangerous because they are poorly integrated and weakly controlled. Is psychosis an organic disorder or is it caused by the attitude of the mother who does not allow the child to become autonomous? Whatever its origin, this pathology leads to the persistence of the narcissistic fusional state in which the imagination prevents the functioning of psychic authorities established during the course of normal development, authorities that serve both to progressively separate mother and child while keeping the imagination at bay. Thus the psychotic, immersed in the narcissist fusional universe, is characterised by an extreme dependence on the fantastical representations which he has forged of his mother, father, indeed of all the partners in his life. He can live, for example, psychically fused to the fantastical image he has of his parents, which will keep him captive in the realm of his imagination, and which are miles away from the reality of his actual parents. His affective relations are fusional and ambivalent; they refer to 'two mothers' in a potent mixture of love and hate.

According to psychoanalysis, the psychotic is in a state of fusion called, in Lacanian psychoanalysis, '*jouissance*' (which is no way a synonym of joyfulness as one might believe: it rather indicates a state of confusion between subject and object). Not possessing an 'outside', the psychotic experiences fantasies which he cannot externalise. He remains a prisoner to an archaic lived experience in which he cannot distinguish outside and inside, imagination and reality, the other and self. He therefore has a disturbed relationship with reality, involving a poor ability to understand relationships, structures and causalities (even if they sometimes manifest flashes of insight and intuition, such as the hero of the film *Rain Man*).

The system of classification of the North American school of psychiatry called DSM IV distinguishes several types of psychosis also included in the psychopathological classification adopted in Europe.[1]

Schizophrenia

When the deformation of the reality concerns not only thought but also perception, this results in schizophrenia; an individual hears voices and talks to invisible people. This disorder is characterised by a shattering, dismembering and dissociation which infect language itself. Words liberate themselves from things and wander without signification as fragments of broken and heterogeneous language resulting in strange, sometimes poetic, associations.

Delusional disorder

Deformation of reality may concern thought, as we see in paranoia with its well-known forms: delusions of greatness and the delirium of persecution or jealousy. The paranoiac interprets everything in terms of his own subjectivity; he is at the mercy of the projections which induce him to endow the other with his own desires. Melanie Klein demonstrates the homology between the paranoid position of the young child (centred on the fantasies of persecution by partial 'bad objects') and the paranoia of the adult.

Joseph, who was 18 years old, arrived at his dance-therapy session in a terrible mood. He had made a scene in front of his girlfriend because she had left a present outside his front door. Confusing the exterior and interior of his apartment (itself a representation of his own body), because he could not distinguish his own inside and outside, he interpreted as an intrusion what, for his girlfriend, was a simple mark of affection.

Other disorders

These include:

- Shared delusion disorder: *folie à deux*.
- Psychotic episodes: temporary delusional episode, post-partum psychosis, delusional mania of bipolar trouble – previously called maniac-depressive psychosis where the unity of the subject shatters and begins to oscillate between two extreme states of maniacal excitation and profound melancholy.

Autism

Another neurobiological condition usually diagnosed during childhood and frequently encountered in dance therapy is autism. Those with autism do not respond well to the outside world. They remain, instead, enclosed within a 'bubble'. According to Melanie Klein, the autistic child takes refuge like this because he has 'burst' from fear or rage. The autistic child will spend their time contemplating objects without ever playing with them. Jerome, a 13-year-old who was attending dance-therapy sessions, lost himself in fascination with a book, pencil and ball. In his passive ecstasy he could not make the least impact on the object. He was incapable of catching or throwing it, just as he was incapable of imitating it. It was as if he felt the 'call' of the world, without being able to 'respond' to it.

How can we incite Jerome to take a step further? How are we to help the psychotic exit this fusion? How are we to enable him to distinguish inside and outside, to separate himself from the other to become the subject of his acts and speech instead of remaining captive to his early fascinations? What are the processes normally employed by the child which we, in turn, should invoke in therapy to lead Jerome out of his imagination, which sometimes takes on a terrifying aspect?: in those moments, for example, where he fixes his fascinated gaze on the mouth of his mother, leading to hours of crying, bashing his head against the wall, or hours seated on the ground turning incessantly in circles without being able to calm down? How are we to endow him with the capacity to free himself from the fascinating image through its replica and to find a living link with the world? In a word: through rhythmic practice, inspired by the work of the mother in helping the baby to differentiate itself from her body.

Note

1 For the European systematic classification of mental illnesses and their etiology, see Bergeret, 1974.

7 Between two

During the course of normal development, the human being retains elements inherited from the period of fusion; yet he does not allow these to overwhelm him. Even when ecstasy remains an integral element of his way of life, as in primitive societies, he remains neither fixed nor paralysed, but rather an active partner in the world. This transition is rendered possible by the creation of a common space shared between mother and child where they 'play together' and where their actions, reactions and playful interactions initiate the process of differentiation.

Intermediary space

At the start of the child's life, where outside and inside are mixed, the Other, thus the mother, is both external and internal. How does the human being, confounding these two realities, the one objective and the other psychic, manage to unravel them, to distinguish the two poles and attribute to them respectively the Other-outside and self-inside, external reality and internal imagination? This is accomplished progressively, under the effect of a double impetus: mother and child, outside and inside, reality and fantasy. Between them there is established a zone of exchange, an air of common production where they play and create together.

Through such activity the child will start to bond with the mother while recognising this 'other', which is to say become capable of differentiating itself from her, distinguishing its imaginary productions from objective reality and keeping thereby its fantasies at bay. Yet even as an adult, the human being will conserve, ready to hand and capable of reactivation, a privileged place where imagination and the world meet and exchange. This is an intermediary space where fantasy and reality mix in common productions through playful and artistic activity.

The mother–child relation experienced through the body

The first relation to the mother is one of total dependence. How could it be otherwise given the pitiful state of the psychomotor capacity of the newborn human? Yet the mother, if she is healthy, will know how to induce the child to separate from her. In order to recreate and adapt, for the purposes of therapy, the autonomising experiences which she offers her child, let us examine her role in more detail.

According to Henri Wallon, the first communication between mother and child takes the form of a tonic dialogue. The baby, living in physiological and affective symbiosis with her, takes part in her emotions through the medium of the body; the very form, amplitude, frequency and rhythm of the movements of the child are based on the maternal response. The postural space of the infant is rooted almost in the literal sense of the term in that of its mother. We have already spoken of the maternal imprint at the corporeal level. According to Wilhelm Reich, Alexander Lowen, Arthur Janov and the neo-Reichean current, the emotions of early childhood are firmly located in the 'body memory'. They can be reactivated, giving access to the first experiences of the relation with the mother and reconnecting the patient to the archaic lived experience of childhood. This is the point of departure for the 'new therapies': bio-energy, primal scream, vegetotherapy, massage, 'rebirth', and so on. Yet if therapy's true aim is to achieve de-fusion, then we must propose to the patient something more than an archaic regressive commemoration. We must take inspiration from the way in which the mother interacts with her child to exceed the passivity of the imprint and to elicit an active response which aids in the process of liberation from the perspective of fusion. For this, we require an intermediary creation.

Psychoanalysis insists on the process of de-fusion by stressing two essential aspects of the role of the mother, two mechanisms for the construction and autonomisation of the subject which we re-appropriate in dance therapy: the construction of the psychic envelope; and the role of the gaze in the shaping of the body image.

By virtue of its non-unified state, the child is invaded by its emotions, which are dispersed without organisation: he must succeed in containing them. It therefore seems dangerous to liberate the archaic emotions of psychotic or autistic patients if we do not also give them the wherewithal to reorganise and integrate these 'dismembered' emotions within a coherent whole. So, let's continue to follow the mother's example. Her communication and interaction with the child possess the double function of activating drives through forms and 'containing' them in these very forms. The gestures, smells, voices, speech and songs from the early experience of the child enable it to contain these experiences by giving them 'moulds'.

The mother plays a crucial role, according to Didier Anzieu, in the process of the psychic creation of an 'envelope' enabling the constitution of a 'self containing psychic contents through the experience of the surface of the body' (Anzieu, 1985: 39). This envelope at first presents itself fantastically as a 'common skin' reuniting the mother and the child in the dyad. It creates a common, rhythmic space in which two 'partners' exchange smiles, movements of the head or hands and diverse vocal productions. We appropriate this structure in dance therapy by establishing a common space where therapist and participants move and chant together by following a rhythm originating from the outside: from cultural heritage or from the repertory of modern dance or popular tradition.

The envelope is the creation of what the mother sends back to the child of the sonorous and gestural productions which the child emits. It matters little which of the two initiate this process. What counts is the reciprocal reflection of these forms, which will come to function as sonorous and gestural containers. Primitive Expression puts its faith in the parallel between the development of the child and the therapeutic process. The movements of Primitive Expression accompanied by vocal productions (of non-signifying phonemes such as the 'language of the spirits' of shamanic rituals) are carried out at the same time by therapist and the group of participants (or single patient in the case of individual cures).

Françoise Dolto, a famous child psychoanalyst, insisted on the importance of the gaze reflected between mother and child. She was able to detect and sometimes indeed to treat certain early autistic troubles by 'working' the visual contact with the very young whose gaze remains vague, never fixing on the other person. By tuning in on the gaze of the child, she was able to re-establish the communication which had faltered at an earlier stage.

Psychoanalysis stresses the importance of the gaze which the mother fixes on the body and the performances of the child, who constructs its 'body image' in communication with this maternal gaze. If the gaze is 'absent', which might occur if the mother is depressed, it awakens emptiness and gloominess. When welcoming and positive, the child engages in vivifying interaction with her. The gaze therefore has the capacity to produce a negative body image when imprinted with bitterness and disappointment (e.g. if the mother wanted a boy but had a girl) or jealousy (e.g. if she is envious of her son).

Replaying the relation to the mother in the transfer of dance therapy

We know that the therapist activates in his patient a 'transfer', which is to say a repetition through the person of the therapist of childhood feelings. Reliving past situations is a key therapeutic tool. It enables us to recreate and re-experience, under the best possible conditions, those situations which had pathogenic consequences, such as an inability to relate to the surrounding world, focusing in particular on the gaze to positively re-orientate these situations. The rhythm dance therapy which we practise is founded on this principle. It reactivates the conditions of the archaic experience in a number of ways: through the sonorous foundation of percussion evoking the beating of the maternal heart; through the non-verbal relation incarnated by rhythm and the chanted voice; and finally, through the structure of symmetrical gestures which is discussed below. The goal is to induce a regression, enabling thereby the mobilisation and intervention of different structuring mechanisms in the early relation, principal among which is the therapist's gaze and its impact on the patient.

In the re-actualising through dance therapy of the situation in which the gaze of the mother was of crucial importance, transfer plays a key role. This allows the patient to reactivate emotions felt in the first relationship with the mother (e.g. dependence, love, the search for approval, fear of judgment, mistrust, or even hostility). To play an authentic structuring role, the gaze of the therapist must be living and attentive: never malevolent. It must be encouraging, positive, approving, confident in the possibility of progress, involving and happy without, however, effecting blissful happiness. We are thus called upon to analyse our own counter-transference, what our own gaze reflects onto the patient. Vigilance towards the risk of counter-transference (i.e. the unconscious emotions which the patient awakens) is indispensable: they can inspire disgust, contempt, hatred or even an admiration which is equally unfavourable to the construction of the patient's self-identity.

We should recall that this therapy is an adapted pedagogy. For the patient, it is not just a question of remembering but of self-reconstruction. Our goal as practitioners of Primitive Expression is not to plunge the patient back into fusion, but to help him to extract himself from it. If, therefore, we aim to reactivate an archaic lived experience, it is neither to cause the patient to lose himself in it (we have one day to leave behind regression, as the infant must leave the maternal bosom) nor for the 'cathartic' effect involved in reliving former emotions. Without neglecting the importance of giving such emotions the possibility of release, which is at the core of Reichian therapy, we insist, rather, on channelling them. We associate the work of the liberation of the drives to the creation of the missing envelope, proposing forms capable of 'containing' the affects and employing both the emotions activated in the patient by the transfer and our gaze as tools in the positive reorientation of the body image.

Jerome, an autistic child of 13 (we met him in Chapter 6), was content at the start of the cure to passively listen to rhythm and percussion, without wanting to connect his motor capacity to it, simply for the pacifying effect which it had on his agitation and anxiety. He remained in apathetic fusion: closed off to imitation, a prisoner of hypnotic fixations; absent in his 'bubble'. We thus attempted to establish communication with him by using percussion as accompaniment while singing a lullaby to him. Immediately his closed expression disappeared, his gaze cleared and he gave us a magnificent smile. This was repeated in each session through the use of rhymed chants, lullabies and nursery rhymes. These served to establish a space in which our first exchanges, both vocal and motor, could take place, enabling a therapeutic relationship to develop.

Transitional space

The mechanisms which enable the cultivation of autonomy, based on the harmonics of the gaze and establishing a relationship (to the mother in the case of the child, to the therapist in the case of the patient) are rooted in the intermediary zone. In psychoanalysis, this is known as 'transitional space'.

Winnicott calls the space between two, the space of encounter of mother and child, reality and imagination, the place of passage between exterior and interior, 'transitional space' (Winnicott, 2005). It is here that inside and outside, fantasy and objective world, self and Other, represented primordially by the mother, interact and create together. Winnicott also speaks in similar terms of 'transitional phenomenon' to designate the mechanism which serves to realise this passage and 'transitional objects' the means by which to accomplish such a passage. We have already observed that, for an object to possess a transitional function, it must evoke the mother (e.g. possess the characteristics which make it loveable – the fluffy softness of a teddy bear or a blanket).

The transitional object *par excellence*, according to the psychoanalysis, is the breast. To understand how it can aid the process of separation, we should remember the child's feeling of being fused to its mother with whom it constitutes a single being, while latching onto parts of the body which psychoanalysis names 'partial objects'. The breast is an example of such an object. It is so intimately associated by the child to its perfect complementarily with its mouth cavity that he imagines that it belongs to him, and he is under the illusion that he has a magical control over it. He believes that he can 'create' it on demand, because the mother produces it precisely where and when he wants it. Winnicott calls this breast a 'transitional object' belonging neither to mother nor child, neither inside nor outside, neither fantasy nor reality. The mother progressively disabuses the child of its fantasy of control, showing that the breast is not under the child's all-powerful influence, but actually belongs to her. Little by little, this cultivates an acceptance of reality and a separation between the two. According to Winnicott, transitional objects are those which invoke the presence of the mother by functioning first as decoys, creating the illusion of her presence and re-creating the universe of fusion. However, they then progressively, help the child to detach itself from this universe. The transitional objects, which have existed for as long as humanity, allow the human individual to articulate its bond with its mother through activities and within spaces which bear the character of 'transition'. They function within a zone shared between two; a paradoxical place since it belongs without contradiction or conflict to both inside and outside, imagination and reality, other and self.

Francis, a 16-year-old psychotic, preferred to 'steal' the recording of the percussion and take it home with him. His mother telephoned the day clinic where he was being treated to tell us about this. She added that he had been masturbating while listening to it. This indicated that the sonorous foundation when employed alone maintained a state of fusion (both with his mother and therapist) and that he used it as an auto-erotic object. There was no 'Other' in Francis' world yet. We therefore asked the mother to bring the cassette to help with the process of separation.

Transitional creativity

Human existence constitutes part of the All, the cosmos: its relation to Nature (the Other) is comparable to the relationship of a child to its mother. The individual constitutes part of Nature without being her. He is bound to her, homologous to her (the microcosm of a macrocosm); he nevertheless differentiates himself from her in becoming her partner, a situation in which each one can exchange with the other.

The permanence of transitional space

The process of separation between the interior world and reality is progressive and ongoing. Realised normally by all individuals during the course of their development, it creates strata within the psyche which remain active throughout the life of the individual and participate in the being-in-the-world characteristic of *homo sapiens*. In fact, the mechanisms through which the fusional 'bubble' is progressively overcome are not subsequently abandoned: each one remains in place and adopts a precise mode of functioning. The most archaic strata are not by any means the least worthy of interest. For example, the imagination is a product of the persistence of transitional space despite being, by definition, 'erroneous'. It is different from reason and is a crucial aspect of human creativity and artistic creation. The complexity, diversity and creativity of human thought result from the interaction between earlier and more recent functions. 'Primitive thought' is continuously being interwoven with 'rational' thought, contributing to the 'genius of the species'.

According to Winnicott, play, theatre, art, religion – in short, all cultural productions – are manifestations of transitional activity. They have their roots in the imagination while at the same time allowing us to escape from it by expressing it in an intermediary space where it can be held at a safe distance.

The transitional objects of dance therapy

The gestures of dance therapy can be understood as 'transitional objects'. They are invested with meaning by both the therapist and the patient, and are an expression of the poetics involved in the construction of the subject. Dance therapy uses rhythm, gesture and voice as transitional objects for their artistic and therapeutic value.

The rhythm of percussion is also an 'object' and plays an essential role. While it functions as a 'maternal decoy' enabling a regressive plunge into the sonorous ambience of the womb, it also participates in the transitional object. Both external and internal, it passes between therapist and dancers as it might between mother and child engaged in a collaborative, playful production which is given/received/reflected by each one of the two partners that it 'envelopes'.

The repetitive gesture is proposed to the dancer by the therapist as it is proposed to the child by the mother. It is then appropriated by the dancer who sends it back to the therapist and so on. This is a process driven by all, as much by the participants who receive and reflect the gesture as the leader who proposes it to the group. As a bifacial, enveloping product of both parties, it continues to establish and maintain this space shared between two: the therapist represents the mother who gives the 'good gesture' at the correct time and the dancers who, by desiring it, create it where it is absent, just like the child.

The emission–reception of the voice is likewise reversible when the therapist and participants in unison sustain a rhythm flow of repetitive phonemes ('Hou' – 'Hou' – 'Hou', for example, or linked and melodic such as 'Oyemaye'). While the therapist initiates the dynamic in that he 'sends' the initial model, the therapist receives the sound which is sent back to him by the group through sustained repetition. A space unfurls in which each one reflects the other.

The intermediary space, zone of encounter and exchange, implies a double movement of two partners, a place of encounter in which emission and reception are reversible. The transitional space is not only a surface, but a space-movement in which the child and mother encounter and reflect each other infinitely in a vital, living relation. We could compare this centrifugal and centripetal dynamic to a kind of 'original dance' through which the child will escape fusion and exist as an autonomous subject.

The rhythm dance therapy of Primitive Expression reconstitutes this transitional original 'dance' by clearly marking the two poles as interchangeable: the repetitive movements initiated by the therapist (as was the case with the shaman) circulate between him and the participants and, because they return identically, reflect each other and create an envelope. Dance therapy enables the patient to escape from fusional passivity, to become the agent of a transitional game, by using mechanisms which solicit the use of rhythm in an active way, mechanisms in which movement and voice are employed as transitional objects 'at the right moment' by the therapist.

Transitional creativity serves as such to prepare for veritable autonomy.

Repetition in rhythm dance therapy

While the fusional fascination is hypnotic, ecstatic, immobile (as, for example, in autism) and the identification passive, repetition leads towards an active form of pleasure: the initial form copies and recopies itself infinitely without end. The mechanism of repetition inherent to humanity appears from very early in life in childish language, 'Areu, areu, areu', 'ta-ta-ta-ta', or 'ma-ma-ma-ma', 'pa-pa-pa-pa', creating the outline of the first names given to parents.

Repetition is a mysterious phenomenon. Does it correspond to the ritual function we have already seen at work in the animal world: the deflection of certain actions towards ends other than their initial goal, followed by their repetition so as to be better 'heard' by their addressee? What function could the insistence on re-commencement have for the human, if not that desire is without limits and supports life? When the child repeats its movements, which seem to re-commence on their own perpetually renewed initiative, it activates a fundamental mode of behaviour whose range of application we have yet to determine. Does it search the pure pleasure of the repeated discharge, or a better mastery of the movement by seizing it at its point of emergence and following its course? Could this mode of behaviour be an epigenetic mechanism seeking to establish a link between inside and outside by uniting them through the gesture, as if each repetition offered the individual another opportunity to latch onto the exterior form? In any case, in its association of desire, pleasure and necessity, the presence of this mechanism is marked in the child who rejoices in hearing the same stories told, the same songs sung, the same game played, and incessantly repeats the same act (e.g. throwing his hat, pulling on a rope, constructing a tower then breaking it). According to Freud, repetition is the 'motor' of the drive, its 'daemonic' mechanism (to the point, indeed, of deceiving death by continually resuscitating action or, in other words, desiring life). He considers it to be so fundamental that he situates it 'beyond the pleasure principle'. It also serves, according to Freud, as a defence mechanism against trauma: an attempt to exceed and re-orientate trauma by repeating it, as in those dreams which repeat night after night the same scene.

Repetition does not always succeed in liberating us from the hold of the imagination, as is clearly shown by the stereotypical activities of psychotics who repeatedly bash their head against a wall or follow the same circuit through a hospital. Repetition can be indicative of failure to exit the All of the undifferentiated. Yet if it is correctly guided by the mother (or the therapist), as a fundamental psychic dynamic which feeds on the instinctual, repetitive corporeal dynamic propelling towards humanisation, it is the first step towards this exit. Should we not see in the drawings of autistic children, who frequently sketch rows of cars and interminable series on varied themes, an attempt to exit the enclosure rather than as 'obsessive' (Figure 7.1)?

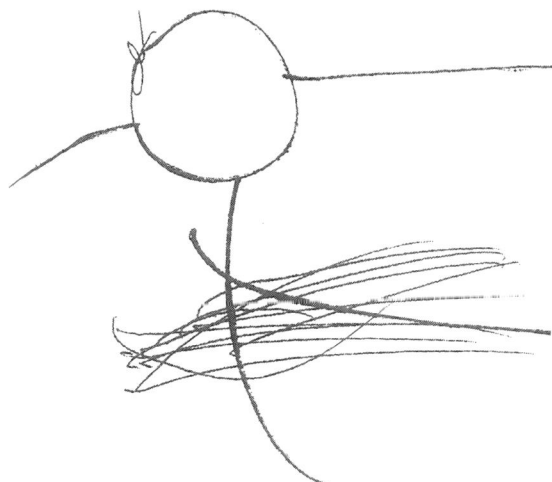

Figure 7.1 Drawing by an autistic child aged 9, after one year of dance therapy, at the moment at which he began to exit fusion. The child could not yet speak (except for a few words) but explained, through a movement of the hips, that he was representing himself dancing. The drawing shows a marked improvement of the corporeal schema: the arms and one of the legs are attached to the body (even if it is to the head). The movement is represented by multiple lines, illustrating the repetition of the swaying movement.

If correctly managed, repetition can be creative and differentiating: the thing repeated is never totally the same, neither in its form nor in its signification. How are we to make sense of this mysterious alchemic transformation which takes place at the heart of the repetition of a movement: a process which, by reproducing the same, creates difference? As Julio Cortázar put it: 'it is strange that people should believe that to make a bed is always to make a bed, that to shake hands is always to shake hands, that opening a box of sardines is always and forever to open the same box of sardines' (Cortázar, 1978). Such reflection echoes the experience of the dancer: repetition inserts into the movement each time a slight difference: a 'more'. It also allows him to grasp that the reproduction of movement proposed 'from outside' does not confuse the dancers within a single identity; it rather encourages each individual to invest his own meaning in the movement. What comes to the fore once the therapist, after communicating the gesture, withdraws behind repetition, and is affirmed with ever greater strength in the movement which returns, is the call of the world searching to reawaken the desire of the subject. It is also the response of the subject to this call, the emergence of the desiring subject manifested in dance through the gesture which represents him with growing force and precision. Let us observe a group of traditional dancers who are all performing the same movement. Such a scenario differs from the arrangement of the Russian ballets where the model is reproduced by all in perfect unison. The tribal dancer interprets the movement in his own individual way: modifying its form, intensity and dynamic; investing it with his own particular character. In Primitive Expression, the recording of the dance allows the individual to perceive this personal re-creation of gesture. This helps to heighten self-awareness and lays the foundation for the therapeutic process.

In addition to its exhilarating character, repetition plays a double therapeutic role in the process of differentiation and the cultivation of autonomy:

- It aids in the destruction of the hypnotic object, the shattering of the fascinating 'One' which blocks the emergence of the subject. Once the body is no longer held captive by the image, it can escape from its passivity.
- Across the 'distance' thus created, the repeated forms 'search out' the dancer as if to invite him to play. Increasing in intensity with each return of the gesture, they 'strike' with ever greater insistence on the threshold of his being, as a messenger knocks on the door in order to be heard.

The parallel with the role of the mother is evident. She emits and the child, face to face, repeats. She also offers the child the possibility of hearing itself vocalise as the dancer, through his movements, feels himself act. Child and dancer are thus able to discover themselves by linking to their own action, in a repetition which is also a return to self.

The advantage of repetition is the pleasure. Exultation is a key component of Primitive Expression and is felt as much in the moment as retrospectively through the recording. The participants, on observing their gestural expressions, are often made to wonder. Paul, an adolescent and psychotic, on seeing his performance on screen following a session exclaimed 'Was it me who did all that?' before adding 'I really enjoyed it!' The surprise is often visible, even if not directly expressed, among the participants who glimpse for the first time the resonating of their body. The encounter of the subject with this reflected gaze on his own experience induces, through the repetitive gesture and a heightening of enthusiasm, an awakening to the plenitude of existence.

Repetition, if it occurs within the context of a living relationship, triggers a deep enthusiasm: the possibility of liberation, a faculty for engagement with all being and of reaching out towards an ideal, a dimension of transcendence whose necessity has been shown to us by shamanism and which we appropriate in dance therapy. The gesture is proposed, offered by the therapist as an action to repeat, explore, enjoy and in which to take joy. Yet the patient is not left alone to accomplish this task. It takes place in the transitional space shared with the therapist in an exchange which serves to cultivate autonomy. We might take, for example, as a point of departure the stereotypical movement of a psychotic patient. The therapist absorbs and repeats this movement, while modifying it sufficiently to avoid giving the impression that he is merely copying it. The patient discovers his reproduced gesture and repeats it. Both at first perform the gesture simultaneously and then alternate. The movement evolves with repetition, becomes progressively more expansive and conscious. The therapist then proposes an action which the patient absorbs, repeats and appropriates. This was the case with Paul, age 20, a schizophrenic, who did not speak but who incessantly raised his left elbow accompanied with a hoarse vocal emission 'Gluff'. This movement was repeated in amplified form by the therapist while dancing, who also added an 'Ou'. Spurred on by the dynamism of the exchange, its repetition and the climate of trust which it cultivated, Paul added his right hand to the movement and amplified the gesture. He became progressively more capable of acknowledging the forms emitted by the therapist and his evolution towards openness, exchange and communication was rapid. At the end of one year, after sessions lasting between fifteen to twenty minutes once a week, he had lost his 'tic' and spoke normally to other people in the institution. This simple and effective measure had only one precondition: the repetition, as in primitive dance or children's games, must be executed in a spirit of sharing and of pleasure. Once this condition was in place, repetition enabled the splitting of the patient–therapist dyad through the creation of a differentiating double, similar in nature to that created by the child in the repetitive games shared with the mother.

Duplication

This process has, as a point of departure, the fusional mimetism which induces the child to echo the actions of the other with whom it identifies. The child is at first in a state of osmosis, crying when the other cries, laughing when the other laughs, etc. This touching sympathy arises in reality from their non-separation, which is the reason for the simultaneity of the two actions. Yet the mother, through this mimetic process, will introduce an alternative dynamic of imitation which will permit the de-coupling of the dyad.

84   The humanising process

The process of separation is long and results from the interaction of multiple processes. They have their origin in the world of fusion where the acts of identification of the child to his mother (and vice versa) serve as the means for their subsequent differentiation and progressive de-fusion. We appropriate such mechanisms in dance therapy, and will now look at some of those which are most frequently employed.

Echo

One example is the echoing of the mother and child through smiles, vocalisations, etc. In the universe of the dyad, enveloped in a common skin, the two partners contemplate and reflect each other in the simultaneity of fusional imitation. Yet the slight delay in the response of one of the members of the couple to the other introduces an initial distance between the two. It is across this echo-like repetition that the possibility of uncoupling the two parties of the dyad can be glimpsed.

In Primitive Expression, yet also in the education of normal children, the performance of the 'hero' always meets with success. A participant stands face-to-face with the group and proposes a motor sequence accompanied by a sonorous emission. We can understand this in terms of the non-verbal enacting of a 'story', acknowledged by the group when it echoes each element of the gesture. The other participants, invited in turn to carry out this performance which consists in transmitting a gestural and vocal production, lose themselves in the pure corporeal pleasure of imitation.

Alternation

The form emitted by one of the two partners of the dyad and echoed by the other is in turn recognised and re-emitted by the first. Smiles and vocalisations (('Areu', 'Areu') are exchanged from one to the other like a ping-pong ball. Such echolalia and echopraxies produce a circular reaction which initiates the exit from the state of fusion without, however, establishing a transitional bridge between inside and outside, the self and other. As such, they prepare for the recognition of the existence of the other (in the word 'alternation' is there not the root 'alter', the other?). Each one takes their turn to vocalise or perform the gesture. The voice and maternal gestures respond to those of the child, while repetition of the phoneme or movement of the latter at first takes the form of an osmotic mimetic response, before understanding that it is the agent of these actions face-to-face with another agent. Firstly fusional, then transitional, the gestural and sonorous forms become vectors of separation. The child succeeds in differentiating itself on the basis of such mimetic, corporeal and vocal games, a source on which dance therapy draws. The following represents an example of an alternation established between participants and the therapist:

- the group, accompanying their voices with a striking movement of their feet on the ground, chant on each fourth beat 'Hou' – 'Hou';

- the dance therapist, on the three remaining beats, chants a melody which weaves between the 'Hou' of participants -'a ya é' – 'o yo ha' – 'bou sa ma' – 'sama yé', etc.

The call of the world

We have seen that repetition embodies the insistent call of the world addressed to the subject and allows us to distinguish the mechanism of alternation from the simple mimetic echo. There remains the question of the source of the child's desire to reproduce it for his own account. Should not the 'mother good enough', according to Winnicott, not precisely renounce being 'too good' to aid in this process of leading the child towards the outside through plays (Winnicott, 2005)? This dynamic engenders the centrifugal and centripetal dialectic in the young monkey who little by little frees himself from his attachment to his mother's fur to explore the world, while returning to bury himself in it during moments of distress. The human child can only cultivate its own identity following its psychic separation from the mother, and it is on the basis of the 'invitation' addressed to it by the exterior world that the child constructs itself as a subject. It is indeed difficult to say who initiates the process: the child, in whom the exploratory drive develops or the mother who awakens it. How does the human child become aware that the world calls it 'lovingly': first through the performances of the mother, then of the surrounding environment which, at first existing in a state of confusion with the child, becomes the double of the latter? This attractive force is perhaps, once again, the result of homological resonances which Noam Chomsky considers to be innate to man, either 'engrammed' at a very early stage or genetically encoded. His fascination for them would therefore be the result of a kind of awakening of an inside element by a 'bringing into phase' with an element from outside. In this Chomsky is in agreement with Piaget, who asserts that the child is capable of interiorising situations with which the outside world presents (in 'epigenetic' fashion as the scientists would say), thanks to the existence of pre-established motor neuron structures which constitute schemas of action (i.e. general patterns that can be reproduced). Whether or not this is true, what is clear is that this call initiates for the child the process of de-fusion and a new type of bond with the outside world on both an affective and intellectual level – levels which are profoundly interwoven. Piaget compares this foundational de-centring of the human subject to a 'Copernican revolution'.

We are led from here onto the plane of a certain dynamic. The development of the 'invoking' drive (as Lacan puts it) insofar as it emerges from the call of and to the world, is driven by biological instinct, an oscillating movement of coming and going between the outside world and the state of fusion.

Copying and echoing

At the level of pre-linguistic games, interaction involves replication in a double sense: the response and the reproduction of the same by replaying it. By receiving from the child spontaneous vocal and gestural forms which she then reflects back, the mother introduces a spatial and temporal alternation. The interaction is established across a mutual echoing: each one waits for the other to send back what they emitted; this creates the two nodes of the dyad.

Unlike the paralysing hypnotic relation, the amorous resonating in phase with the world renders the child active on the motor level. The process of imitation ceases to involve the passive absorption of the model, engendering an intense desire to create its double. At around the age of 1, the vital need to reproduce the forms of the environment makes itself felt. Furthermore, through the concept of 'assimilation', Piaget sets out the character of sensory motor intelligence. This is an intelligence which is essentially practical, founded not on concepts but on movements, and which the child activates through the repetition of actions from reflexes to habits to imitation. Aristotle had already asserted that man is 'the most imitative of all the animals'. According to Marcel Jousse, this is because he internalises the forms of the world (its centripetal call) and replays them corporeally (the centrifugal response). This enables him to pursue the process of decoupling between the world of fascinating forms and himself, passing from fusion to partnership (Jousse, 1974).

Dance employs the same mechanism: a form comes from outside and awakens (enters into resonance) with the self. It thereby incites the desire for movement which is a powerful tool of de-fusion. All traditional dances, whatever their origin, play this double role, making them transitional activities *par excellence*. Their rhythm renders them 'maternal' by invoking the rocking and swaying which recall the fusion with the other, yet also 'paternal' insofar as they awaken the desire to exit the confines of the self to engage in action. The gestures which they propose satisfy the contradictory aspiration towards both the ecstatic dimension and autonomy: by virtue of their dynamic character they are able to straddle all such opposition, to instil in the dancer the desire to seize, mime and play with them.

A comparative study of such dances has yet to be carried out. Are there forms which, in a universal way, call for a motor response? If so, do they draw on fundamental rhythmic and gestural structures? Do they evoke archetypal figures? Under what conditions do they carry this double function: both reassuringly 'maternal' and dynamically 'paternal'? Whether universal or not, it is abundantly clear that the power of attraction of such dances is a constant across civilisations. It is relatively easy to recognise the therapeutic movements in traditional dances (by allowing oneself to be seduced by them) as they present the paradoxical character of transitional objects: both 'resonating' in the imagination and 'opening' towards the exterior.

Rhythm dance therapy takes inspiration both from the shaman and the mother, using the 'objects' of popular dance, with the firm conviction that their collective gestures, whether from Europe or beyond, harbour the ability to awaken vital forces and to re-organise disorder.

8 Gestural symmetry coupling with the other

It has become ever more common among psychologists to see a parallel between the work of the mother leading the child towards individualisation and that of the therapist accompanying the patient towards a state of autonomy enabling him to live in a less alienated and chaotic way, humanised by his relation to the other. To this end, the rhythm-dance therapist helps the patient, just as the mother helps the child, in applying symmetry and harmonics in his relation to the world. This encourages the patient to initiate a non-verbal dialogue through alternation, establishing a link with the Other in its capacity as a singular entity no longer submerged in fusion.

Escaping from the state of fascination with the world does not prevent the child from remaining in solidarity with it. He can take part in the world while differentiating himself from it. To communicate with the other, he must discover that he is someone and not a mere component part of the other.

The mother–child dyad embodies an incomplete scission whose partners find themselves separated/united in an oscillating movement which binds them joyously together.

Symmetry in rites, games and dances

The importance of symmetry both in dance and in other fields is largely recognised in traditional societies. It has been celebrated in rituals since Antiquity (Daraki, 1994: 87) through swings (e.g. in Greece, where it is still practised today in a number of cultures). They offer the opportunity to corporeally and joyfully relive the operation which links two distinct partners in an oscillating movement of mutual recognition which lays the foundations for human existence.

We observed two brothers of 6 and 3 years old playing on a swing. It was the opportunity for them to create couples, associating verbally at times their two first names and at others 'papa' and 'mama' or 'pappy' and 'mammy', tirelessly repeating and subsequently recombining them in diverse ways. The youngest cried 'Christmas'! with great enthusiasm each time the seat was launched towards the sky, then remained quiet on the journey back down, as if the second movement of the swing required silence in relation to the time of flight exulting towards the sky of 'Christmas'. Was he thus associating 'sky and earth', the supernatural and everyday world, the Other and himself?

In this oscillation, the movements of climbing and descending are bound within a binary couple: ascension precedes and announces descent, which itself serves as prelude to and announces re-ascension, and so on. The binary movement, therefore, involves the pleasure of anticipation, already encountered in repetition. What is more, it carries with it the vertigo of automatism: of a perpetual, autonomous movement back and forth, creating thereby two entities which are inseparably linked. When the swing is at its height, the child knows that it is going to come down again without intervention. The swinging, therefore, induces the abandonment of movement which takes hold of the body. It is beyond the control of the latter; the self finds itself unmanned by the intoxicating dynamic which both fissures and binds two people and two worlds.

Dance celebrates the origin of man by supporting structures of rhythm, repetition and symmetry which reactivate in the dancer the harmonics involved in such childish games. The captivation of the body by this movement cultivates positive emotion through the feeling of being rocked and swayed by an 'Other'. While it is included today only hesitantly, or in veiled form in ballet, both modern and classical, it is at the core of tribal dance. It persists in traditional dances of the folk variety and is resurgent in the current trends (swing, groove, rock) of popular dance.

The dynamic sources of gestural symmetry

Such symmetrical forms of movement issues from the lived experience of our own body, whose essential dynamics are harnessed by and becoming the carriers of fundamental significations.

Symmetry as a genetic mode of behaviour

The child discovers symmetrical forms of movement very early (rotating the head from left to right, and then later on all fours moving back and forth), which very possibly correspond to genetically programmed modes of behaviour already at work in the animal. The baby practises such movement, particularly when its mother is absent; it allows him to feel a sense of security. René Spitz recounts that children whose mothers display excessive forms of behaviour, alternating rapidly between explosions of anger and demonstrations of tenderness, frequently appeal to binary movements, as if to unify the contrary attitudes by endowing them with their own logic. Swaying may also constitute a stereotype, a compulsive behaviour characteristic of psychosis. We meet it frequently in hospitals and psychiatric institutions in children who oscillate part or all of their body in a sterile and desperate fashion, enclosed in a world without any opening and failing to create the other.

The archaic relation to the mother

These movements echo the maternal practices we saw at work above: the rocking of the child in its mother's arms or in the cradle, the alternating from one pole to the other of the dyad through the vocal or gestural productions of the mother in response to those of the child, the rhythmic and tonic dialogue of their relation, and so on. In all such dynamics we see a binary exchange between two partners emerge in an exodus from the state of fusion. We might indeed say that all such symmetry, from rocking to games of imitation, seek to appropriate the practices employed by the mother in bringing the child to the recognition that the two are both separated and united in a dynamic bond.

The corporeal foundations of gestural symmetry

The elements brought into play in such dynamics are above all those which the morphology of the human body provides.

Verticality and symmetry: the cross

The biological heritage of evolution has endowed the human with received physical characteristics which serve as the basis for his psychic development. By standing up, he puts himself in the plane of verticality which distinguishes him radically from the animal. This verticality succinctly expresses, in symbolical terms, his condition as the union-rupture between earth and sky which, in turn, become two primary signifiers of his bipolarity along with human world/divine world, mother/father, body/soul, material/symbol, etc.

Aegean civilisation has left us with numerous archaic statues dating from the third millennium BC depicting the human being standing straight with arms spread, the body in the form of a cross as the product of two intersecting lines: the trunk as an axis of vertical symmetry and the arms horizontal symmetry (Figure 8.1). If the verticality of the body allows it to become a signifier of the union between sky and earth, the separation of its two halves signifies its division, the rupture between the Other and self. The doubling of the dyad is transposed onto the shape of the body in a process indicated by the fashion in which the single foot of the statuettes is split into two adjoined feet. At the same time, the horizontal bar of the arms outstretched symbolises the 'horizontal' relation to the other human, the one who resembles us. We will adopt for its clarity and simplicity the distinction established by Lacan between the Other, which transcends man (the dimension of the symbolic, culture, language, God) and the other (fellow humans, the first among whom is the mother).

The vertical and symmetric figure of the cross reaches to the essential nature of human existence. Symmetry implies a body made of two halves connected along a median line. Yet the frontal representation of the verticality of the body and the symmetry of the two sides is not evident at the outset. It must be conquered and integrated into the corporeal schema.

90 *The humanising process*

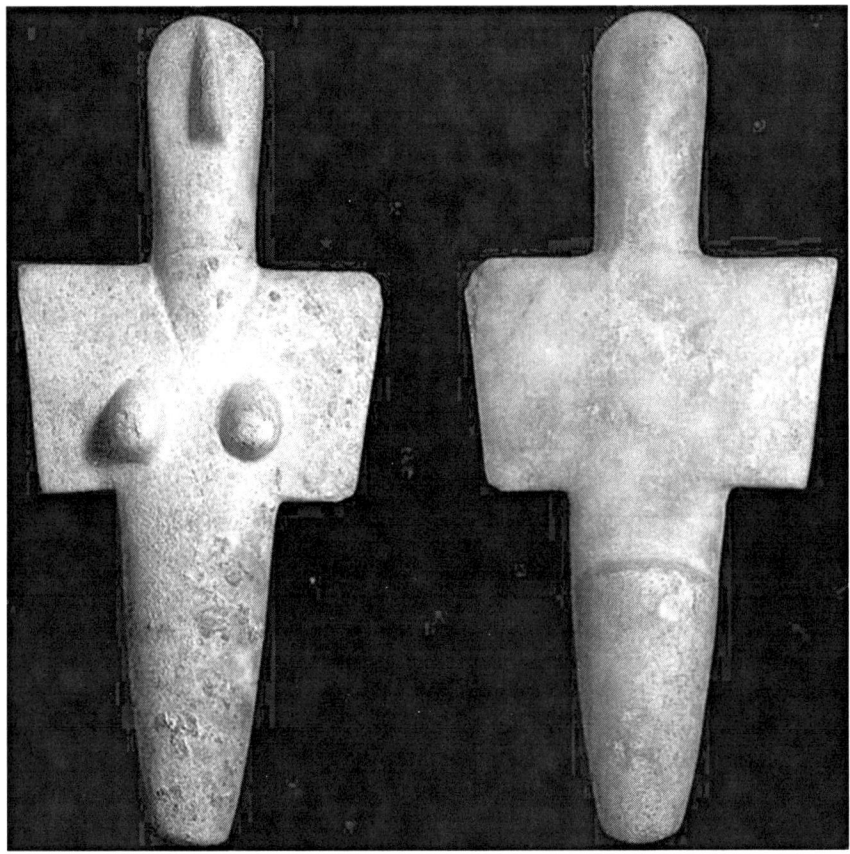

Figure 8.1 Cruciform figurine, 3000–2500 BC
Source: J. Paul Getty Museum, Los Angeles

Verticality is the embodiment of force, a resting on sure foundations. We perceive it, above all, in the vertical axis crossing through the body, a rising vector aligning the vertebrae into a column which supports the body and frames the self (Anzieu, 1985: 98). We insist on verticality in Primitive Expression from the heels to the tips of the fingers, arms stretched towards the sky. Verticality constitutes for the body image an interior skeleton which appears, in the drawings of children who exhibit normal development, in the form of a cross (Haag, 1985: 107–114). It is, moreover, a favourable prognostic when it is drawn by certain psychotics at significant moments of their cure (as we shall see below).

Bipedal movement

The perception of the separation of the two feet, together with the acquisition of verticality, leads to the movement of walking, another founding element of humanity. The locomotion of man takes place exclusively on the lower limbs and all the weight of the body, when vertical, rests successively on each one of the two feet. The two sides of the body are each called upon, in their turn, which implies a lateral swinging of the trunk. At the same, an oscillation backwards and forwards, which is particularly visible in the arms and pelvis, is required to re-establish equilibrium.

Gestural symmetry in dance

If our peasant dances or the dances of 'primitive' societies, have persisted and attract much interest today it is because they were developed over the course of centuries from the perspective of the community, not the individual. As a result, they carry embedded within them, in their music and gestural behaviour that which most essentially characterises the human species: its morphological and psychic laws. They transpose, onto a different level, the transitional steps we all, as individuals and as a species, were obliged to take in our path towards humanisation.

We dance standing up, expressing the verticality of the *erectus* in which the feet interfaces with the earth and the head is attracted towards the sky. Rural, 'primitive' or 'traditional' dance is intensely relational: we do not dance or sing alone but in a group, in relation to the other, to others, to music. It offers the pleasure of dancing together, of sharing a collective resonance and a gestural code common to all in the group. Finally, they are constructed according to the logic of the bipedal body, which possess its own inherent gestural harmonics. 'My feet, my dancing mad feet!' (Nietzsche, 2003: 243) exclaims Nietzsche who saw in such symmetry and harmonics the very essence of dance. Dance unfolds in time and in space. With regards to the former, a rhythm of two beats governs perambulating motion: the two feet striking the earth, in turn, for equal duration. In terms of space, the continuous left-right oscillation of the walk serves as the basis for a range of symmetrical movements which alternate from one side to the other. That the rhythm is in two time (2/4, for example) or in three time (6/8) matters little: what counts is that the movement remains poised between the binary poles of a dynamic which synchronises the different members and in which the body is engaged in its entirety.

We might say, in general terms, that the harmonics of the body involved in symmetrical, oscillatory movement back and forth, left to right, is the source of rhythm in dance. Bipolarity reigns in both instances. The movement of the dancer splits into pairs (split representation) grouped around an axis, whether vertical (from left to right) or horizontal (from high to low). The two half movements constitute a couple in the same way that the unity of the body in bipedal motion emerges from the left and right hemi-corpus.

In primitive tribal dances and in a particularly marked way in Primitive Expression, the coupled sections, whether rhythmic, sonorous or gestural, are shorter than in traditional dances. Their step and movement are punctual and repetitive. This renders them more accessible and easier to perform – indeed deceptively so – because they harbour other challenges. If the sequences of movements are rendered briefer through deconstruction, they are also rendered more expansive and intense. Their energy, which increases with each repetition, leads the dancer little by little to a state of forgetfulness of self in a voyage to the exterior world, culminating in a state of trance in which he or she is entirely possessed.

In the collective movement of the group, the dancer forms part of a collective subject. The 'I' becomes 'us'. Each individual constitutes part of a greater body with several heads and twice more legs, yet with a single heart: that of a rhythm which is both sonorous and gestural. Yet even if the dancer is part of a body, if the relation to the other is above all collective in that all dancers are on the same level and share the same sentiment of belonging to the group, the dancer remains very much an individual and his imagination in a waking state engages in dynamic meditation. The dance speaks differently to each one, and his creativity pairs them in its own unique fashion. The coupling of pairs of movements, complementing those of the feet, creates a bipolarity: the two symmetrical movements become partners alternately occupying centre stage. In company with Nietzsche who feels the 'intoxication of opposites', and with the child who cries 'Christmas' when the swing is at its height and falls quiet when it falls back to the ground, the dancer accentuates unevenly the two poles of the binary movement. In rhythm, the high time names itself 'strong' time, and the time of withdrawal 'weak' time.

There is, indeed, encoded within the act of walking an affective differentiation to the alternating of the feet or different phases of the movement which renders the movement signifying. Creativity is, however, a secret mechanism and the meaning invested in the movement is untranslatable. Nobody knows quite what it signifies, not even the dancer.

Bipolar movement is a metaphorical expression of fusion and separation. One foot, for example, represents the Other, the outside; while the other foot represents a return towards the self. The binary step enables a life which alternates between the two states, establishing thereby a dialectical relation to the Other. This could explain *a contrario* the robotic, mechanic character, of the march of numerous psychotics, which has not yet come to signify the couple 'I-Other'.

Restoring the link

Gestural symmetry unifies the body, synchronising all its parts from the feet to the head and counteracts the feeling of dismemberment. In primitive dance, a double bodily axis, a line of sharing, of both unity and division between two twin entities, structures and brings them into resonance. It is not content with unifying the body. It connects, by pairing within binary couples, all the essential forces which determine human existence: the mother, the other, the self, the group and the cosmos in a joyful relation of reciprocal echoing.

When the link to the exterior world fails, resulting in pathology, the appeal to structuring binary movement such as that offered in rhythm, dance, music and poetry constitutes a powerful therapeutic tool. Rhythmically timed gestural symmetry, the repetition of couples, both creates a double and binds this double according to a bipolarity. This is true whether we are speaking of the two halves of the body, the self and other, two components of the self, or finally self and absolute Other, as in the case of the mystics for whom the body becomes the vehicle for entering into union with God.

Binding the two sides of the body

Observations of children in conjunction with clinical data show that symmetry is not present from the outset in the constitution of the image of the body. The fantasy of the dismembered body is often expressed (e.g. in autism and psychosis) in terms of the sensation of the two halves of the body not being 'stuck together'. Dance allows us to create a unified body image by experimenting with the movement of the body with a view to installing symmetry: we 'feel' in turn each hermi-corpus and connect them through an alternation of a bipolar, 'binary' rhythm which pairs them in space and time.

For the baby, who experiences its body as dismembered, such integration must be acquired. Geneviève Haag, psychiatrist and psychoanalyst, has carried out extensive research into the corporeal junctions at work in the development of the child (Haag, 1985: 107–114). She observed that, when the mother is absent, even if only for a moment, the child will pacify itself by joining together certain parts of the body: not only, as everyone knows, thumb and mouth, but foot and mouth and the two hands and feet.

Haag's observations are in concordance with the representation of the human body in terms of a cross. Its vertical bar corresponds to a stylisation of the vertebral column. The appropriation of this axis implies the existence of a suture uniting the two halves: indeed the interior skeleton appears as a cross in the drawings of many of the children who undergo treatment. To Haag, this figure seems 'to bear witness to the process of a profound integration . . . the installing of a kind of internal skeleton, the corollary of a psychic skin sufficiently solid to enable autistic detachment as well as the attenuation of pathological symbiotic phenomena'.

In those cases in which the cycle of repetition has not been broken, and a binary exchange between two poles has not emerged, dance therapy can intervene.

The body image of Florian, 11 years old and psychotic, did not possess a left side. Suffering from no neurological deficiency, he could nevertheless only execute movements to the front or to the right. He was incapable of immediate imitation. He lacked one of the terms for bipolarity, as much in his body (the left half) as in his relational life where the possibility of recognising and echoing the other was absent. Yet unbeknownst to us, he would practise it later, imitating the therapist long after the session had finished. We became aware of this when one day his nurse, who accompanied him to the sessions, repeated the movements of Florian on the platform of the metro as she was taking him back home. To our amazement, he had correctly reproduced the dance of a monkey, elephant, clown, soldier, using both sides of his body, which he then accomplished with ease during subsequent sessions. His case seems thus to demonstrate that temporal oscillation, even when occurring across some considerable time, provides the foundation for a link of alternation between therapist and patient, one necessary for the union of the two sides of the body.

Haag cites the case of an 8-year-old child who, because of his inability to use the left side of his body, had initially been diagnosed as hemiplegic. During psychotherapy sessions, he would draw by 'sketching interminable series', which instead of writing off as 'obsessive', I believe should be interpreted as an attempt to pass from repetition to the creation of a dyad. It is, in effect, the absence of the integrated structuring of such a dyad through symmetry which prevents the construction of a unified body image among seriously psychotic or autistic subjects. This helps us to understand their anxiety at being 'badly stuck together'. Let us recall that, as Freud stresses, the 'sick' show us in minute detail the psychic structures of the 'normal'. Haag, indeed, recalls a question which she was asked by a little boy exhibiting otherwise healthy development, yet suffering from somewhat strong primitive anxieties: 'are my buttocks stuck together properly?'

Working on the hypothesis that the autistic or psychotic pathology is linked to the non-integration or disintegration of the two halves of the body, we harness the unifying and integrative function of dance therapy to mobilise and bind these disparate halves through the dynamic of alternation, an example of which we have seen in the case of Florian, The integration of the capacity to link with the other manifests itself in the child as the development through repetition of paired gestures of a gestural harmonics between the left and right hemi-corpi, according to an axis of vertical symmetry, or sometimes between top and bottom, according to a horizontal symmetry. The child reproduces in both cases the split representation of the movements at work in primitive dance. We will observe how such dances, by contributing to the constitution of two poles, enable an escape from psychotic fusion. Their dynamic reconstructs the archaic history of the human individual by allowing the possibility of incorporating the dyad. It engenders the existence of an exterior connected to an interior, an exterior which is thereby no longer menacing (let us recall once again the young monkey leaving and rediscovering the maternal fur). The dancer finds himself thus capable of alternating between two distinct temporalities: time of fusion and time of separation; centripetal time and centrifugal time; time of the self and time of the other.

By transposing into culture a fundamental stage of his or her development, the process of coupling in a movement of gestural harmonics, the dancer invents a cultural form of therapy, one which is capable of detecting and healing a troubled body image indicative, as we shall see, of a fault in the link to the mother, the first other of the child. It is in these terms that dance has functioned as a favoured means of prophylaxis and therapy throughout the course of human history.

Internalising the primitive link to the mother

Haag arrives at the conclusion that each side of the body represents one of the entities of the child–mother dyad enveloped by a common skin. This implies, in similar fashion to cellular biological division, a division within the interior of a single membrane. The child reconstitutes this totality by integrating the two halves of the body. This will allow the child to separate from the first 'half', the mother, by internalising it: which is to say, the external 'other' first enters the human being in corporeal terms. Gestural symmetry creates two poles for the Other (the mother, but also the exterior world, nature and culture, in particular language): an Other located both outside and inside, constitutive of the subject according to an identity which has become dynamic. If we follow Haag, whose clinical observations led her to assert that the two sides of the body function as analogies for the two members of the dyad, infant and mother, the body becomes homologous to this dyad insofar as the relation between the two halves incarnates within the structure of the body the first relation to the mother. We should further note that the two halves of the body, shared between the maternal (or paternal) function and the child, are not necessarily mapped against the vertical axis of the cross. Its horizontal axis can serve the same role, such as can be observed whenever the child performs the habitual gesture of putting its foot in its mouth.

It would appear therefore that the body incarnates the bond between the child and mother in an analogical way: the left side seems more often to represent the primary half (as was the case with Florian) and the right the secondary half. Observations on babies of five months have shown that the right side serves to ensure security through the flexion/rhythmic extension of the leg, while the left executes modes of behaviour such as gripping and the grasping of food. Similarly, the left thumb (which represents the baby) plants itself in the cross of the right hand (which represents the mother), and so on. Inversely, the failure of the differentiation of the couple mother–child finds expression among autistic children in the joining of both hands which clasp each other with such force that they can only with difficulty be prized apart, a clear sign of the persistence of fusion.

Specularity and the constitution of the self

The autistic child is unable to establish a link to fellow humans and is similarly incapable of harmoniously linking the two halves of its body.

The apprehension of the self as an entity of two halves is at the core of our self-identity: a development to which the mirror stage is essential. With the mirror, of course, it is not a question of the anatomical symmetry of two halves, but a communication between self and its 'immaterial double'. The result, however, remains the same: the division/union of the individual through which he becomes a whole while remaining in two differentiated/interwoven parts. The very term 'oneself' suggests that it is by way of the detour through the double that the individual apprehends himself, according to an identity constructed in dialectical relation to the matching 'Other' glimpsed in the mirror. He is bound to this image, though he is not it and it is not him. This quandary lays the basis for the task of decoupling at which Narcissus and the psychotics fail. They remain fixed in a time prior to the constitution of the mirror stage, and are unable to construct their specular identity, the reflected totality, which allows the child to perceive itself as separate from the body of the mother. How, then, are we to lead them to this structuring articulation of self to self?

Application in the treatment of psychotic and autistic patients

If the integration of the two sides of the body serves to interiorise the link between mother and child, and thereby between the I and Other, we may suppose the efficacy of psychomotor practices which reunite the two sides, such as primitive dances. I use the rhythmic movement of primitive dances performed in synchrony with the therapist to recalibrate the foundational relation to the mother. The hope is that the reactivation of the link to the mother, through homology to such rhythmic movement and through transfer to the dance therapist, might serve positively to re-orientate it.

Haag's observations on the identificatory integration of the mother–child relation via the two halves of the body corroborate my own observations made during the course of therapy. Like Florian, psychotics and autistic patients often use only one half of their body. It is not rare, for example, for them to follow rhythm with either the left or right side exclusively. While capable of repetition, they are unable to escape from it to participate in a game of two. Their auto-erotic rhythm involves a single term incessantly repeated. Everything happens as if they had not discovered the means to activate the second term, which would allow the Other to emerge.

It is for this reason that we propose to them movements such as the opening and closing of the arms and legs, or a succession of symmetrically opposed actions, such as concealing the face behind the hands before allowing it to reappear. Seated in front of the patient with or without the support of an external rhythm, the dance therapist holds him by the hands and rocks from side to side, transmitting this movement of oscillation accompanied by an opening/closing of each hand. The certitude involved in the reclosing of the hands, guaranteed by the insistence of the rhythm and the security which the therapist provides, is often sufficient to coax the patient into temporarily releasing the 'life buoy' which the gripping of the hands represents. Through the use of such movements, we have several times induced psychotic children to unclench their 'fusional' hands. In Cyril's case, I was able, through the same means, to induce a hand–mouth relation which is often lacking among autistic children. The movement of the hand towards and away from the mouth, to a rhythm shared by the couple therapist–patient, served to establish a link between the two parts of the body and assisted greatly in cultivating in Cyril the ability to feed himself.

With these pathologies, Primitive Expression uses a multiplicity of rhythmic, symmetrical movements in parallel with a diversity of musical styles (e.g. traditional and contemporary music). The goal is to cultivate a dynamic between participants of which the following are some examples:

- A game of echoes established between therapist and patient, each one producing and reproducing in turn movement and voice. This creates a

spatial and temporal alternation, sometimes distended as we saw in the case of Florian, but always establishing a link on the model of the game played between mother and child where each repeats the other.
- The performance of symmetrical movement serves to internalise the link to the therapist (to the other) through the joining of the two halves of the body and the establishing of an oscillatory exchange from self to self.
- The exchange of gazes between patient and therapist: the gaze, in fact, does not imply a unilateral dynamic between watcher and watched. There is an economy between active and passive roles, which could well be an important factor in the constitution of the specular image. Knowing that the body image, which determines to a large extent the image seen in the mirror, is influenced by the gaze of the other, we sometimes record performances to reinforce the link between the self and its image. Dance therapists frequently observe that the relation of the self to its own image viewed through the medium of the recording retraces the path which leads the child to the constitution of specularity. Its image in the mirror at first appears to the child as other, unrelated. In similar terms, the participants filmed during the session are invited afterwards to watch themselves on the screen. Their first reaction is a feeling of foreignness: they declare themselves troubled and fascinated by their own image as before the apparition of a 'double' which is not them. Following the example of the child, they will have to 'domesticate' their image to bond with this double and represent themselves through it.
- The binary character of the voice accompanies that of rhythm and movement. The pairing of sonorities or words is a fundamental mechanism, one which drives, for example, the functioning of the unconscious. The mobilisation of vocal harmonics therefore gives us access to the most profound levels of the psyche, and is of clear benefit to any therapeutic framework.

The therapeutic treasure of oral cultures: bilateralism

In rhythm dance therapy, the coupled forms used are present and still living in oral cultures. Each one of us conserves, engraved indelibly in his memory, the rocking movement which brought sleep and the lullabies or songs shared with other children. The almost ineffaceable character of their presence in our brain is derived from this rhythmic link: each half of the verse awakens the other which matches it and replies by mirroring it in terms of duration (the same number of 'feet' as in the alexandrine or multiplication table) and sonority (Je l'attrape par la qu_eu_e/Je la montre à ces messi_eu_rs).[1] This coupling through melodic, rhythmic and phonetic analogy corresponds to what Marcel Jousse calls 'bilateralism': the translation into the symmetry of language of the symmetry of the body (Jousse, 1974).

The harmonics of bilateralism

In similar fashion to gestural symmetry, all vocal sequences seek to find a matching partner with which to form a couple. The homologies we have encountered in the context of shamanism and the world of symbols are nothing other than such paired terms. Bilateralism can be seen at work in the primary processes of the unconscious magical formulas, poetry, music and dance and the primary processes.

It is indeed through the medium of the primary processes that the human body and the world are bound together. The primary processes are the ensemble of mechanisms which constitute the 'Id', the reservoir of drives and the pleasure pole of the unconscious. Their rhythm animates the functioning of what we might call 'primitive', 'savage' or 'pre-logical' thought, which represents the world to itself according to the couples which are at the foundation of all modes of thinking, even the most complex (Lévi-Strauss, 1966). This linking of homological entities through a semantic harmonics known as the 'association of ideas' could indeed be defined as the 'dance of the unconscious'. Anchored in its oscillatory dynamic, they are responsible for the apparently absurd character of its logic which assembles things not according to relations of cause and effect (linear logic) but of analogy. Such analogies might be based, for example, on form (the serpent and the penis), colours (blood and jasper stone) or homophonies (rhymes), rhythmic sequences (songs and lullabies) or indeed the coupling of opposites (angel and demon). The primary process can be recognised in childish language, creating 'absurd' associations through games involving phonetic doubles: the repetition of consonants, vowels, syllables, words and phrases. Such doubles can be found in all childish songs:

> Tombe, tombe, tombe la pluie
> Tout le monde est à l'abri
> Sauf (e) mon p'tit frère
> Qu'est sous la gouttière
> Qui pêche du poisson:
> Pour toute la maison.[2]

The paired words are linked through the symmetry of their oscillation as much to the body as to each other. This is indeed the reason for the ease with which they are memorised, as well as their 'magical' influence on each other.

They are also at the origin of the dream and of its strange associations, as well as of word games which pair unusual elements. This use of wit results in laughter when confronted with rational thought because of the fashion in which it puts elements into a relation which logic finds entirely incongruous. The unconscious, which obeys its own logic, is not shocked by this and in 'literal' fashion translates ('converts') into corporeal terms one of these elements, a process which results in bodily symptoms. A number of psychosomatic troubles are of this origin. An asthmatic patient enjoys repeating 'I did everything for my mother', a phrase which in his unconscious phonetically and rhythmically resonates with another: 'I suffocated for my mother'.[3] A woman who is allergic to fish discovers the confusion, made when she was a child, between 'fish' ('poisson') and 'poison'. Problems of the 'knee' are frequently the corporeal translation of a difficulty involved in articulating together the 'I' and the 'nous' and so on.[4] Everything happens as if the body had made a spelling mistake which is, in reality, a game played between the initial phrase and its homophonic double.

Magical formulas

This capacity of association to anchor and thereby 'convert' linguistic terms into bodily terms explains why its procedures are used in magical-religious operations (e.g. ritual, prayer, sacred formulas or enchantment).

Here, for example, is one of the formulas employed by the 'fire healers', traditional healers who are still called today to heal serious burns:[5]

> Feu, feu, perds ta chaleur
> Comme Judas perdit ses couleurs
> En trahissant Notre Seigneur
> Dans le Jardin des Oliviers (Loux, 1979: 144).[6]

Association is, in addition, at the core of artistic expression: not only music and dance, where it is particularly evident because it takes possession of the body and expresses itself through it, but also in plastic expression; and particularly in poetical expression.

Poetry

Poetry is the realm of binary movement. It swarms with homophonic similarities which couple elements which at first sight seem foreign to each other. Lamartine offers some interesting examples of this:

> Le soir ramène le silence
> Assis sur ces rochers déserts
> Je suis dans le vague des airs
> Le char de la nuit qui s'avance.[7]

Poetry pairs the objects of the world. It also pairs these objects and the self in relations of binarity whose strength is drawn from the bodily rhythms which they incarnate (thus the significance of the prosodic term 'foot', which reminds us that poetic verse was initially accompanied by the striking of the feet on the ground).

Drawing on this ability of association to link two terms in a doubled and twinned identity, poetry possesses the 'magical' power to transfigure the objects of the world. It knows how to create an association which reveals mysterious correspondences between things and transforms the world into a densely woven tissue whose binding element is human existence. Association is an act of love: the self weaves together forms which also weave themselves; whatever is capable of forming a couple is married with passion. Poetry not only associates man and the kingdom of all living things, it also associates the elements of the cosmos which enter into the universal play of resonance. Poetry creates the frame for a canvas which includes the living and inanimate world, the cosmos and the poetic self thus coupled with the world: the Dionysian man of Nietzsche who feels the happiness of existing as a participant in a living, single substance (Nietzsche, 1999: 113). Binary movement is the instrument of this poetic continuity which represents not only the mute fusion of a hypnotised man, but also his dance with the world.

Rhythm dance therapy uses poetic images whose dynamising force, a direct effect of symbolic efficacy, is immediately evident. We also ask participants to create 'raps' in small groups which express in poetic fashion an aspect of their problem.

In one session, a group of young adolescents who had held an animated discussion about their mothers' forbidding them to go out in the evening, and of their desire to disobey, composed and choreographed the following 'rap':

> C'était un petit chat tout blanc
> Qui avait quitté sa maman.
> Il est parti en conquérant
> Elle l'a laissé en sanglotant
> Mais quand il aura appris la vie
> Il reviendra lui dire merci.[8]

Two years later, these young people remember with pride this rap which had reinforced their feeling of belonging to the group and eased their relationships with their mothers.

The world of sympathies

Binary movement is not exclusively corporeal;[9] we cannot separate the psychic and somatic: it includes all existence in its sweep, in an amorous coupling (*syzygique*) of human existence with the universe. It is profoundly linked to the elements of Nature: such movements form with her an ensemble of dyads which constitute totalities. The feeling of participation derives from the paradox of a unity of substance emerging from the splitting of existence between the two great paired entities of the cosmos and the play between them, a couple which interact in similar fashion to the twins whose lives seems constantly to influence each other.

The pairing of man and the cosmos is poetry incarnate. A human being is bound with nature through a network of correspondences, affinities and sympathies which weave a common fabric and are at the foundation of the 'animistic' feeling of taking part in the All: Nature is the 'macrocosm' which doubles the 'microcosm' of the human body. This pairing allows us to understand the concept of symbolic effectiveness, the scientific name for magic. Let us note that 'primitive' beliefs do not necessarily disappear with the advent of modern technology: since the Chaldeans, astrology has put man and the constellations into shared resonance by proposing correspondences between the signs of the zodiac and character traits, supplying it thus with a means for acting on the body and creating analogies between the constellations and different corporeal zones. This analogy is at the root of the efficacy of the symbolic system of healers who still practise today in rural France (for whom Taurus is said to govern the neck due to the size of the bull's neck, while Gemini governs the 'twin' entities of the shoulders, etc). The associations which pair the universe and human existence determine the so-called magical practices at the heart of popular and traditional European medicine. The coupling of agate with milk, for example, is in reference to the martyrdom of Saint Agatha whose breasts were cut off. The strength of their sympathy is such that as soon as we interact with one of the two elements, we act at the same time on the other. If the jasper stone stops haemorrhaging, so the rock of agate produces milk in a woman.

It is from interactions such as these that the symbolic potency which we observed in traditional therapies emerges. Abandoned in the West by biomedical discourse, it nonetheless obstinately persists in numerous practices of 'soft medicine'. It is only to be regretted that the latter are held captive by a pseudo-scientific discourse which renounces the symbolic origin of their effectiveness, which is to say the sympathy (the homologies) which connects man to the world which surrounds and pervades him.

Notes

1 'I catch it by the tale/I show it to these men.' The homophony between 'queue' and 'messieurs' is, of course, lost in English.
2 'Fall, fall, fall the rain/Everyone is under shelter/Except my little brother/Who is under the gutter/Who is going fishing/For all the house.'
3 The play on words here, lost in English, resulting from the consonance between 'J'ai tout fait pour ma mère' 'I did everything for my mother', and 'j'etouffais pour ma mère' 'I suffocated for my mother' (translator's note).
4 The French for 'knee' is 'genou', or 'je-nous': 'I-We' (translator's note).
5 Such symmetrical, harmonic movement can also be observed in the contrasts and rhythms of the most complex compositions.
6 'Fire, fire, lose your heat/as Judas lost his colour/while betraying the Lord/in the Garden of Olives.'

7 'The evening returns the silence/Seated on these deserted rocks/I feel the waves of the breeze from/The chariot of the advancing night.'
8 'There was a little white cat/who abandoned his mother/He left triumphantly/She sobbed as she watched him go/Yet when he has discovered life/He will return to thank her.'
9 We could, perhaps, extend the coupling phenomena to the recent discovery of quantum physics. Two electrons, brought into contact with each other, remain implicated subsequently by virtue of their 'spin' magnetic orientation, if we separate them and we change the spin of one, the other, even at a distance, will reverse its own spin. At the moment, we are not able to identify the nature of the link which creates this effect.

9 Bilateralism as structuring dialogue

In the game of seesaw which can be found in parks all over the world, two children seated at the two extremes of a plank alternatively rise and descend. One might say that the one who is high calls to the other to climb, while, the one who is low calls to the other to descend again. It is a game, in other words, of call and reply.

The pair call–reply

We observe a similar type of dialectic in the movement of walking, with the sole difference that the 'players' are the two feet. A game call–reply transposes itself into the body, since each gesture is in a state of equilibrium with its symmetrical counterpart. All movement of the body precedes, announces and awakens the double which succeeds it. The latter, in its turn, replies and 'calls' the first, and so on. Since each partner calls its homologue, each call awakens an identical response which, in its turn, functions as a call. Call and response are reduplicated to infinity. African dance is a good example of this kind of dialogue: the symmetrical and formally identical movements succeed each other in an infinite call–response through which the body of the dancer becomes the locus of a perpetually renewed dialogue between twin entities. We appropriate this system in its entirety in rhythm dance therapy.

This dialogue between call and reply possesses another aspect, one which also renders it so rich in consequence, particularly in terms of the access to language it opens: reversibility. If the movement of the seesaw awakens the interest of so many children around the world, it is because the reversibility of its dynamics interrogates them so profoundly. One mounts whilst the other descends; the movement of the one finds its double in the reverse movement of the other. The two partners therefore mirror each other: the child observes that the movement of going is the reverse of the return, which is itself the reverse of the going. A 'reversibility' is established between two terms according to which each can be viewed from two contrary perspectives and thus understood in two contrary senses.

Dance likewise engenders symmetrical movements across the axis of the human body, movements which are identical but not interchangeable because they cannot be superposed. They are joined in the same reversible relation as that of the child with its own image in the mirror. This identity differs from that which we observed at work in repetition, insofar as it is expressed through the symmetry of paired movements which present themselves as reversible entities: a reversibility of two opposed and symmetrical directions, determining one as call, the other as reply. This dynamic explains certain aspects of the bilateralism we observed in Chapter 8, whose malfunctioning is at the origin of disorders relating to conversion or symbolic effectiveness.

Finally, we should recall that the two symmetrical trajectories, though identical, are not equivalent on the affective plane. Generally speaking, we go somewhere more happily than when we return from it. This difference in psychic lived experience is in fact at the origin of a distinction between two temporalities. We saw this in the example of the child who cries 'Christmas' in the upward but not downward movement. There is an emotional difference between the 'going', an enthusiastic *élan* towards the exterior (in this case the supernatural realm), and the 'return': which is to say, a withdrawal into the self; a silent, melancholic time whose *raison d'être* is perhaps merely to re-launch the first movement. Implicated in gestural symmetry is therefore also a difference: a 'limp' expressed in binary rhythm through the alternation of a strong and weak time. The stress placed on the first corresponds to the return of the event-pleasure (and by virtue of this, the strong time is what we wait for and is more energetic). The difference between the two moments of the dynamic which gives human rhythm its characteristic 'limp' distinguishes it from the monotonous and uni-polar rhythm of the metronome.

At the heart of the method of Primitive Expression, our brand of rhythm dance therapy, is a vocalisation which enables us to mark the paired movements (or sequences) through a difference in phonemes (e.g. 'oyo é' on the one hand, 'oyo a' on the other).

To stress the foundational character of call–reply, we respect the upper case letters allocated to them by ancient Gnosticism, according to which they become the two authorities, the twin pillars, organising the world, inciting the supernatural (the Sky) and human domain (the Earth) to call and reply to one another. Their divinisation is an expression of the automatic character of their dynamic, embodying a force which acts independently of the human being who indeed remains under its thrall. The joining of the two poles via this dynamic in turn engenders the individual as a fully fledged human being. We will later see how psychoanalysis likewise locates the emergence of subjectivity in the bond uniting the invisible and visible, the symbol and the thing which it designates.

The mechanism of the interaction call–reply stretches to all the couples governing the psyche of man, linking them in a binary dialogue:

- space: the symmetrical paired movements (linking right/left, in front/behind, high/low);
- time: the 'binary' rhythm coupling before/after, night/day, day of work/day of rest;
- relation to other humans: mother/child, subject/other;

- relation to the world: inside/outside, world of nature/supernatural world; and
- physic states: sleep/awakening, imagination/reality, madness/reason, 'right brain'/'left brain'.

The call–reply structure creates an unwavering reciprocal, reversible and symmetrical bond between these fundamental couples, which structure human existence in the world. Once this link is perceived, as it is in dance, the redundant character of the dualism which would separate them in hermetic fashion becomes abundantly clear. We will describe here some other human activities which enable us to live this structuring interaction, and which are therefore particularly useful within a therapeutic framework.

The calling power of archetypes

The uncoupling of reality and the imaginary world is necessary to enable the patient to emerge from the state of fusion–confusion which, though normal for the young child, will, if it persists, result in psychosis. Making this distinction requires a balancing act on the behalf of the child: the outside world and the world of fantasy alternate, calling and replying, awakening and echoing each other. They thus produce a shared, intermediary object, the simulacra, where the worlds of reality and illusion encounter each other. This world corresponds to a 'half-belief', because it is no longer a hallucination, nor yet a representation: it conserves a fragment of the existence of that which it duplicates. It cannot be confused with the object; yet functions 'as if' it were this object. It is transitional, like the teddy bear which 'simulates' the mother by 'presentifying' her through its softness and warmth. Neither entirely decoy, nor entirely distinct from the object, the transitional object is a simulacrum, participating in its reality through the conduit of the 'as if'; a child can incarnate through play an imaginary monster, he believes in the reality of it, yet at the same time he does not believe in it: a paradox which enables him to remain linked to the universe by this 'half-belief' which is both 'inside' (fusion) and outside in the exteriority of the one who is not duped (separation). The arts which 'imitate' reality are founded on the structure of the simulacrum. They invoke the presence of that which they simulate. It is this presence which gives to the simulacrum its presence, power and magical efficacy, known to anthropologists as 'symbolic efficacy'. For example, the images of figurative pre-historical painting constitute less, for their authors, the representations of things than their double.

The force of this interaction is indeed badly served by the term 'imitation', which too weakly qualifies this ultimately hypnotic process in which the original is interiorised, absorbed and appropriated. Marcel Jousse prefers to speak of 'mimism', underlining that the human, and particularly the child, is above all a mime artist. It is through miming, the incorporating of the image or behaviour of a 'model' as its simulacrum, that the human being 'magically' borrows something of its real presence. He is both other, while remaining himself.

Of course as westerners we must ask ourselves a series of questions: Can the therapeutic range of the simulacrum exceed the framework of cultural product? How might we benefit from their power, the therapeutic effectiveness of myth, if we no longer believe in myth? Must one think that their intensity is linked to 'faith'? What is the degree of belief that we must invest in these representations? At stake here is the status of mythology, the ensemble of narratives to which man adheres more or less faithfully. 'Did the Greeks believe in their myths?' (Veyne, 1983), one historian asks, encouraging us in our reflection on the status of their 'truth' to refer to the example of 'Father Christmas'. The child believes in him 'only halfway'; he is poised between two perspectives: he is convinced that the marvellous gentleman comes down the chimney carrying toys for him; yet he also knows that the toys are left by his parents, and innocently sings 'my beautiful tree . . . which Christmas has planted in our house by the hands of my mother'.

The myth, as a both true and false representation of these otherwise inexpressible experiences, can be placed in the category of simulacra. At the same time, however, it opens a second world beside the real world, one which is not content with simply doubling reality. It aims to transcend this first world: to bring an 'other' world into existence, one which is allegorical, a transfiguration of the first. It becomes 'truer than the truth'. To stop believing in this world in the name of reason and science would deprive us of an essential dimension of human existence; yet this is precisely what is happening in our own time. What do we lose in the disillusionment which repeats that of our childhood: the disappointment, revealed to us as a promotion of the 'truth': Father Christmas does not exist?

Is it possible to believe without believing? We will answer in the affirmative. When we embody myth through the simulacra of art, dance, theatre and play we discover our profound and intense link to it. Without doubt, myth conserves something of the fascination and irresistibly convincing character of the decoy. We are both duped and not duped, enchanted by this 'bifacial' register, half-lure half-representation: a transitional space which brings 'magical' activities, 'spaces of illusion' (let us clarify once more 'semi-illusion'), and powerful agents of metamorphosis into existence.

Myths have an impact on the human psyche which is independent of their religious context. We find, indeed, mythical figures and archetypes not only in religious discourse, but also in tales and legends, in epics and popular songs (hero, wolf, sorcerer, fairy, jester, trickster, and so on). Their contents are implicit, expressing themselves through simulacra. We use it a lot in rhythm dance therapy because they do not speak of the 'aggressive drive' but of the 'god of war', a language accessible to the unconscious. From this point of view, myth is not 'false', as long as we do not understand it literally in 'integrist' fashion, but rather in terms of an intuitive, mystical language which poetically translates a reality which is otherwise inaccessible. This indeed finds confirmation in science: the Oedipus myth is invested by psychoanalysis, as in similar terms, the Narcissus myth becomes the bearer of a certain truth.

These 'secular' myths serve the same function as religion: to give form and meaning to psychic lived experience by proposing mythical representations which 'contain' and express them in an acceptable way. The traditional symbolic forms, awakening, channelling and supporting our drives, bringing them to expression, incite us now more than ever to play with them. If we hold to the Freudian idea of a 'memory of the species', an idea which genetics does not contradict, we may indeed suppose the persistence in our genes of the 'moulds of simulacra' allowing us to mime important scenarios in our history: not only primitive scenes, incest and castration; also hunting, duelling, plundering, hostage taking, the triumphal return of heroes, the struggle against the forces of evil, the quest for the Grail, and so on. Engendered in the encounter with the unconscious and hereditary structure of real models, cast within the 'mould' of the archetype (Jung, 1989: 367), such myths give form to our most profound lived experiences, producing doubles of them capable of translating into representations which allow us to express, acknowledge and share them with our 'human brothers'.

In rhythm dance therapy we employ archetypes (warrior, hunter, princess, bird, snake, etc.) which, though they are not divinities, play the same role by allowing the dancer to 'play' with his drives through them. Dance therapy replaces the religious framework with that of art. How different are these two frameworks? In both cases, the rite (religious or artistic) offers not only a representation, but also a way of living and feeling this representation through the body.

Rhythm dance therapy harnesses the therapeutic power of the simulacra: it establishes a space of illusion (group illusion) and employs magic rite (symbolic efficacy), play, theatre, the incarnation of myths and possession. It thereby exceeds the usual framework of psychotherapy to invoke the ancestral, curative, shamanic function of art, using the power of the 'call–reply' bond to obtain its results. This can be clearly observed in the danced forms whose evolution engenders, in a call–reply dynamic with the dancer, the re-creation of the latter.

What of the other associations discovered by the child in its exploration of the multiple pathways across the link between call and reply? We will now attempt to follow the modalities according to which the child activates such pathways. In so doing, we will identify once more the parallel between their emergence during the course of ontogenetic development and their presence in the structures of dance. We will finish by considering the possibilities for their application to dance therapy.

The pairing of opposites

Contrary to what one might expect, opposites form pairs which are all the more solid for being opposite.

The child's discovery of opposites

I had the opportunity to observe the complementary interaction between a mother and her child who was 3 years old. She was playing the classical game of 'now you see me, now you don't', opening and closing the door, first revealing, then hiding, herself. Each time she appeared, the child, who was seated on the couch facing the door, burst out laughing; as soon as she closed the door, the child let out a cry of impatience for her return. The pleasure of anticipation of the child was manifest. During the course of the game, the little boy added his own complementary action which was very interesting. Each time his mother showed herself through the open door, he hid his face in his hands; when she closed the door again, he opened his hands while saying the word 'Go', pronounced in imperious fashion as if to order her to return. Their circular character appeared like the call of each individual to their complementary half: the action of the mother as a reply to the call of her son, a reply which itself was a call for the action of the child.

This exchange between mother and child reproduces in dynamic fashion the profound interlocking of their bodies: they adjust to each other and complement each other. This bond finds expression in the representations of the maternal goddesses and later in the numerous paintings of the 'Virgin and Child' which recasts the archetypal figure of the mother carrying the child on her knees, held against her and completing her like a piece of a puzzle. The two halves of the couple are not identical, yet, through their complementarity, are all the more tightly woven together. When the child begins to differentiate himself from the mother, he will remain intimately linked to her.

We find a similar dynamic at work in the child's wrestling with the difficult question of the difference between the sexes which are anatomically complementary. It is also at work in the discovery of the complementary character of the upper limbs ending in its prehensile, concave instrument, the hands, and the convex extremity of the lower limbs, the feet. Such complementarity, echoing that of the mother–child relationship, permits it to integrate the upper and lower part of the body. Finally, we may suppose that the child recognises the same character in the relation of the two feet in bipedal locomotion, possible only in the harmony expressed when one foot is raised while the other remains on the ground. It is thought that the process of matching opposites is relived and perhaps, indeed, reinforced, by the movement of walking which is homologous to it, the symmetrical movement of the feet alternating in such a way as to create a binary rhythm which is itself also symmetrical. Walking, which appears at the same time as language in the development of the child, is instrumental in enabling it to perceive in the labours of the body the game of call–reply which brings the two feet into interaction in the symmetry between opposed and complementary elements. As such, it incarnates a link made at the point of juncture between all such relations, one which is as inseparable as that of the double.

Once again, *homo sapiens* seems to have used his phylogenetic heritage to gain access to his psychic structure. On the basis of the experience of its relations with other and with its own body, an understanding of complementarity emerges in the child, one which superposes on the game of call–reply a difference which predestines the two entities to a secure interlocking.

Even if the harmonics between call and reply no longer governs the duplication of the same, but the apparition of the different, this difference remains in intimate relation to the original in a play of complementarities.

The human child will relate this discovery to the experience of symmetry (a particular case of complementarity linking two entities along a shared axis) and reversibility, all of which contribute to the production of the totality. The child will also link the complementarities to a search for opposites which has always impassioned it. The repetitive game of alternating between centrifugal and centripetal drives led it from a very early stage to put into repetitive play two opposed actions: throwing the hat away and bringing it back, throwing the ball and bringing it back, opening and closing the door, switching the lamp on and off, climbing up and down the stairs, etc. Understanding now that their coupling is equally a complementarity, one which reconstitutes a totality, the child perceives the indestructible link which binds such opposites. From the age of 2, it experiments with them extensively by setting in motion all sorts of pairs of contraries via a diversity of games.

This period also marks the beginning of the famous 'no phase' where the child opposes itself systematically to whatever is demanded of it. All educators should understand that he does not adopt this behaviour through 'caprice', but to create a new bond to his mother, allowing him to differentiate itself from her by exiting the state of fusion. It is not a question of rebellion, but of reaching towards autonomy and is a sign of health. In initiating this search, the young human indeed embarks on an ancestral quest, as the study of our prehistory demonstrates.

Binary opposites in anthropology

Leroi-Gourhan points out that, on the walls of the Lascaux caves, the paintings of animals do not represent 'hunting scenes', as was previously thought; rather they represent, through the illustration of herds of bison and horses, two opposing yet complementary principles, two forces in interaction: the feminine and masculine nature respectively (Leroi-Gourhan, 1964). This same relation symbolised by paired geometrical opposites can be seen at work in the art of the Magdalenian period (8,000 years BC) and later in the ancient Mediterranean in the form of divine couples bound according to 'syzygies', two married couples embodying contrary and complementary values: the feminine divinity linked to the earth, immortality, love, night; the masculine gods in the sky, youth, death, hatred (Schott-Billmann, 2006: 69–91). Examples of these are Isis/Orisis in Egypt, Cybil/Attis in Asia Minor, Astarte/Tammuz in Syria, Aphrodite/Adonis in Cyprus, Demeter/Dionysius in Greece.

The recognition of the fundamentally complementary character of contraries is also evident in the traditional Chinese couple of yin and yang (Figure 9.1). In a dynamic interlocking of two principles, the feminine yin is associated with wetness, darkness and receptivity, the masculine yang principle with dryness, clarity, activity. Turning back to psychic organisation, let us note, finally, that Freud draws a parallel between the life drive–death drive and the two great physical principles which govern the movement of celestial bodies: attraction and repulsion.

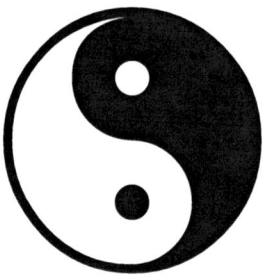

Figure 9.1 Yin and Yang

The human sciences also locate the existence of pairs of opposites in 'savage thought' and mythology (Lévi-Strauss), in linguistics (Chomsky) and in the emergence of the human subject through the birth of language (psychoanalysis takes into account the latter through the child's discovery of the game of opposites culminating in the inaugural 'fort-da' which we will look at later in this chapter).

Without fully knowing why, do we not all feel profoundly concerned by the 'archetypal' representations of the Taoist schema of yin and yang or of the *syzygic* couple of the ancient Mediterranean, or indeed their modern variants such as the icon of Saint Constantine/Saint Helen in contemporary orthodox cults, as if we recognised something essential expressed through them (Schott-Billmann, 2006: 170–182)?

The prevalence of such binary opposites in the cultural productions of humanity, as well as in the development of the child, shows us that we are dealing here with a fundamental anthropological structure. We should not, therefore, be surprised by their presence in primitive dance.

Paired opposites in dance

The putting into play of opposites finds expression in dance by establishing binary movements which follow each other in repetitive fashion. These opposites take on a diversity of forms:

- body (stretching/contracting, round or angular movement . . .);
- space (withdrawing/advancing, moving in a symmetrical fashion from right to left. . .);
- time (slow/rapid rhythm, movement/rest . . .);
- intensity (alternating levels of force . . .); and
- intention (attraction/repulsion, attacking/fleeing, giving/taking . . .).

Setting these into motion unleashes the 'intoxication of opposites' which so fascinated Nietzsche: a call–reply which circulates automatically and incessantly between two movements, leading the dancer to a state of enthusiasm in which he exceeds the limitations of his own self-identity.

It is not a god which possesses the dancer, but the automatism of the call–reply which functions as an autonomous motor. It is as if the body dances alone, as if its movement possesses its own inherent momentum in the perpetual cycle of the call from one to the other.

When this circular motion occurs not within a single body but across two bodies, such as mother and child, it binds them within the structure of a differentiating relation in which each one awaits the response of the other. Dance therapy proposes a multiplicity of such binary games, all of which culminate in the recognition of self and other as two separate entities. For Alexander from Paris, a 9-year-old psychotic, as for Luigi in Italy, an 11-year-old autistic child, treated in Sardinia by Dr Vincenzo Puxeddu, such games led to the exhilarating discovery of the possibility of existing in interaction with the Other represented by the therapist. Since these children did not possess language, the call–reply therapist/patient dynamic was carried out non-verbally by alternating reciprocal imitation or in the complementary pairing of contrasting vocalisations. The former involved musical instruments (the therapist 'calls' with the drum, the child 'responds' with bells), and rhythms which are materialised through the body (the therapist taps with the hands, the child strikes his feet on the ground). In the case of the latter, the dance-therapist Dr Vincenzo Puxeddu used non-verbal vocalisations emitted spontaneously by the child, organising them into alternating patterns, such as the following:

Child: 'Assaoué o',
Therapist: 'Tamata oué',
Child: 'Oôssaoua a',
Therapist: 'Ayamaya hé', etc.[1]

In both cases, a range of different gestural games ('dances') were proposed/received alternatively by the patient and the therapist, involving dynamics of complementarity and 'hide and seek' (appearing/disappearing). Alexander, very apathetic at the beginning of the treatment, one day mimed the 'little puppets' who 'make three little turns and then leave' by imitating the hand movements of the puppets facing each other, before turning in a semi-circle and emitting a barely audible vocal emission. Then, when he restarted the sequence, he laughed out loud, delighting in the alternation between the manifestation and the disappearance of the puppets whose return is already guaranteed. He subsequently made rapid progress showing significant improvement in his body image, which became more fluid and receptive, as well as in his ability to communicate.

According to Winnicott, access to true autonomy presupposes the ability to be alone: to continue to exist independently in the absence of the mother. This implies being able to console oneself in face of this absence, which in turn requires the discovery of the pair Absence–Presence.

Note

1 A therapeutic process applied by Doctor V. Puxeddu in Sardinia in 1991.

10 Symbolisation

The path of the child towards language is long and arduous, since he does not at first perceive his mother as an 'other'. They are fused in the symbiotic totality which lingers from the uterine world. The child exits this fusion via the discovery of the harmonics of gestural symmetry and bilateralism in which the two partners become the double of each other like phonemes of the first words ('ma-ma', 'pa-pa', 'bé-bé', etc.). This process reconstitutes a modified unity based on repetition, in which the mother remains identical to the child. The discovery of alternation, however, leads the child to recognise their differences, not just in terms of the temporal lag of repetition. This is a difference which will extend to their identity, signalling the renouncing of fusion and the aspiration towards autonomy, an aspiration concomitant to the attainment of language.

This monumental achievement requires the discovery of a fundamental opposition made while playing with a diversity of symmetrical oppositions: the couple 'absence–presence', a discovery which will both sow the symbolisation and permit the emergence of the subject.

Descending to the underworld

During the first months of life, the child cannot represent an absent object. We know the observations of Piaget: conceal a toy under the carpet; the child may cry but will not think to look for it. It has ceased to exist for him. One might say that the object only exists as present, as visible. Let us recall that anxiety, said to be 'of the eighth month', which affects the baby from whom the mother has distanced herself. It is not able to symbolise her, which is to say, represent her as absent (invisible). It loses her and sinks into despair. Given that the mother is not yet 'other', is part of him, does he not lose a part of himself? Will she reappear? Nothing is less sure since the child does not have the capacity to imagine it, and thus sinks into anxiety, captive to the persecution of its fantasies of destruction, dismemberment and death. Disappearance remains, for the wholeness of the one who is left behind, an ever-persisting menace in every subsequent experience of separation. Absence is lived as death. It is expressed through mythical language. An example of this is the archetype of the descent into the underworld as a transposition of the experience of the dismembering of the body abandoned by the mother (Schott-Billmann, 2006). There are a number of gods who have had this experience, paradoxical for an immortal in what constitutes a representation in the supernatural register of a specifically human problem. Universally widespread, the vision of the underworld, a dark subterranean and frightening place, full of danger, inhabited by shadows and tortures, superimposes on death (which by definition cannot be represented), the anguishing fantasies which assail the child whenever the mother leaves. Death becomes a place of disappearance without hope of return, an archaic experience shared by all humanity.

How will the child succeed in overcoming the trauma of such abandonment?

The liberating rhythm

In a rather surprising way, grief (the separation from the mother, therefore of the loss of a part of the self), sacrifice (whose fearful character is highlighted by the terrible term castration) and absence are not ultimately expressed in melancholic fashion. They are rather expressed through the exhilaration of play, in front of the mirror or through a rhythmic game. Like the newborn, the psychotic patient exists in a state of fusion–confusion in which inside and outside, imagination and reality, the other and self, are not distinguished. Liberation from this state can be glimpsed, however, in this rhythmic game known as 'fort-da' and described by Freud (Freud, 1981: 10).

It is in play that the child accomplishes the de-centring of the upheaval amidst which the other comes into view and, in the same measure, the self separates from it. This radical change of perspective (which Piaget compares to the Copernican revolution) is acquired through the practice of all sorts of structuring games. To those shared with his mother, the child adds one of his own, essential for its development, dreamt up during the absence of the mother and through which the child 'invents' a meaning in relation to this absence. In the second year of life, during which the child initiates the play of opposites, it discovers the ability to use such opposites to signify the couple absence–presence and apply it to the two 'states' of the mother: when she is there, present and visible, and when she is absent from sight, therefore invisible. The child thus invents activities of the same type as that imagined by the grandson of Freud who gave it the now famous title 'fort-da'. This is how Freud describes what he observes in this boy, aged one-and-a-half:

> The child had a wooden reel with a piece of string wound round it. It never occurred to him, for example, to drag this after him on the floor and so play horse and cart with it, but he kept throwing it with considerable skill, held by the string, over the side of his little draped cot, so that the reel disappeared into it, then said his significant '-o-o-o-oh' and drew the reel by the string out of the cot again, greeting its reappearance with a joyful 'Da' (there). This was therefore the complete game, disappearance and return . . .

The child finds thus the means of transforming an experience of displeasure into a game. In addition, according to Freud, 'an increase in pleasure of another kind, yet direct, is linked to this repetition'. The discovery of a substitute makes us forget the distress provoked by the absence of the mother, enabling the child to separate from her by consoling itself through an object which replaces and symbolises her. The Viennese psychoanalyst, here the attentive grandfather, forwards the hypothesis that the child, by replaying the maternal departure, understands that the reel can symbolise both the mother gone far away, which is the meaning behind the phoneme 'o-o-o-o' ('fort' = far in German), and returning ('da' = here) to her child.

This is the source of the 'increase in pleasure'. This game which at its origin corresponds to a repetition of the trauma of the maternal departure, the loss of real presence, permits the child to win a real victory: the object symbolised can no longer escape it. The child can now conjure in its guise his symbolic mother. The trauma is mastered through its commemoration repeated to the point of intoxication.

The evidence of the structuring importance of 'fort-da' is abundant, and while not every child uses the reel, there is no shortage of such games of absence/ presence: hiding the face behind a handkerchief, which involves the same oscillatory movement of objects such as the yo-yo or ball; the alternating of appearance/disappearance (hide and seek); taking pleasure in running away or waving goodbye, and so on. These numerous and varied devices allow the child to give expression to and thereby tolerate absence, and in the process gain autonomy. The child not only accepts separation, but takes pleasure in it, finding enjoyment in symbolic substitutes put in the place of real protagonists (himself and his mother). It is the game of 'fort-da' which liberates from psychosis, from fusion, from fascinating and destroying the evil eye: from everything which petrifies the horizon of the child, fixing it in place. Distress and anxiety are surmounted. The assumption of subjectivity is a joyful experience. It bursts into the awareness of the child who contemplates himself in front of the mirror or who plays with opposites. From where does this enthusiasm originate? Freud sees in the 'fort-da' the mastery of absence through which the child, by voluntarily renouncing the mother-spool, gains access to separation. He adds that through this game the human child discovers at the same time the possibility of separating from the mother on its own initiative:

> it is from another motive that the child has turned the experience into a game. He was in the first place passive, was overtaken by the experience, but now brings himself in as playing an active part . . . The flinging away of the object so that it is gone might be the gratification of an impulse of revenge suppressed in real life but directed against the mother for going away, and would then have the defiant meaning: "Yes, you can go, I don't want you, I am sending you away myself" . . . It is known of other children also that they can give vent to similar hostile feelings by throwing objects away in place of people.
>
> (Freud, 1981: 10)

Lacan adds a supplementary dimension to the Freudian interpretation by underlining that the 'fort-da' also allows the child symbolically to put himself in the place of the coming and going of the spool. It is therefore the child who, separated from its mother, liberated from her movements, appears and disappears in its guise. The complementary character of the appearance/disappearance of the mother and child we evoked above allows us to understand this role reversal through the dynamic of call–reply. Lacan stresses that the repetition of the departure of the mother causes a division; yet he adds that this is surmounted in the game of 'fort-da', which aims in its alternation only ever to be the 'fort' of a 'da' or the 'da' of a 'fort' (Lacan, 1978: 76). The joy which this game procures is derived without doubt from exceeding such oppositions, and the exhilarating feeling of emerging intact from them. The experience of existing is concomitant to the discovery that in the automatism of the movement, it is the body (that of the dancer or of the child unwinding/winding the spool) which, as the locus of their mutual and reciprocal call–reply, holds within itself and draws together the oppositions leaping from the domain of 'fort' to 'da' and vice versa. In this act of containment and setting into motion, the self is deeply aware that he 'is' his own body as the axis drawing together absence and presence. Thus it becomes the locus for the advent of subjectivity, a subjectivity which thus harbours within itself the Dionysian infinite circularity triggering the feeling of enthusiasm felt in primitive dance. The subject emerges from the movement which permeates him (trance) and which he appropriates (mastery).

Separation from the animal kingdom

The child can recognise himself just as well through non-verbal forms, images, gestures (which differ from simple 'movement' in that they are carriers of meaning), rhythms, melodies, and so on. These substitutes can resemble or take their distance from what they designate. However, the discovery of the resonance of these forms, which is, say, the recognition by the subject of their ability to evoke, is not necessarily supported by a realist resemblance. There is, indeed, a distance between man and the animal. On the basis of graphic creations, such a comparison would allow us to grasp something of the 'revolution' which takes place in the human through the advent of the symbol. Desmond Morris reports the Gardners' observations on the emergence of the capacity to draw in both the ape and humans (Morris, 2005: 111–115). At around the age of 2, both the infant chimpanzee and the child discover with delight the possibility of leaving graphic traces on paper: of producing points, lines and shapes; inventing, exploring and combining. This corresponds to the scribbling stage. They both then strive to create fundamental geometrical forms around 3 years of age, abstract figures such as crosses, squares, circles, triangles, waves, cross-hatchings, etc. (Figure 10.1). The first graphic universe is a world of pure non-figurative forms. Abstractions come first: yet are they 'free' and non-signifying, or already evocative of a reality which both represents and veils at the same time? We are not in a position to come to a decisive response on this question, though we will report nevertheless the reply of 3½-year-old Billy to an adult, who had remarked:

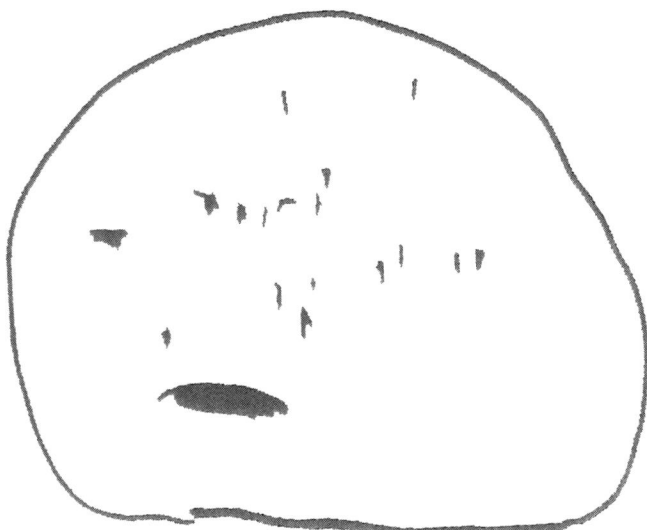

Figure 10.1 Between image and sign: the marked circle, drawing by a 4-year-old child

'I asked you to draw me a bird and a sun and you draw me doodles!': 'You do not understand! I am drawing clouds, the bird and the sun are behind them!'

We could take this response to mean that 'behind' the 'cloud' of abstract forms, the young child glimpses something. It is as if he expected the arrival towards the start of the fourth year, according to Desmond Morris, of an illumination to which the ape is never privy. Via the circle covered with points (a figure called the 'magic circle'), a graphism which is half-image, half-sign, the child, in a veritable insight, discovers – 'invents' – the face which is watching it draw.

It is no longer the pure pleasure of a form which gives it joy. It is no longer the decoy because there is no illusion: the child will not look behind the paper to discover there the real object. The 'true' face is absent and yet exists in its representation. This discovery is the cause of much joy for the young human: he recognises (behind the cloud?) an 'other' who signals to the child from the site of her absence by rising from nothing. The world of forms has taken on meaning for him. It activates this capacity for dazzling evocation characteristic of the symbol.

According to the degree of detachment from the object, the double can function as luring presence (illusion), simulacrum of the immanent presence (image) or invisible symbol (returning to the essence or 'soul' of the thing). It accompanies the process of humanisation signalled by the advent of image and sign.

What is the mechanism through which the human individual acquires the capacity to avoid the decoy of appearance, to 'see behind' the objects, to attain the virtual reality of the object, its symbolic essence? It seems that the body and the rhythm are necessary in the setting up of the 'dance' between absence–presence; that is to say, the liberating dance of 'fort-da'.

The 'fort-da' dance

The game of 'fort-da' is testament to the fashion in which symbolisation becomes rooted in the body. Freud's grandson used several non-verbal substitutes to represent the departure and return of the mother (or himself):

- an object, the reel which winds and unwinds;
- two phonemes, 'o' and 'a', or two opposed sounds, the one closed, the other open;
- two movements of the arm, sometimes stretched, sometimes contracted.

This game, which consists in associating rhythmic and alternating movements, cannot but evoke dance, which once again proves to be the carrier of fundamental humanising operations. This is particularly true of primitive dance in which the state of intoxication induced by symmetrical movement leads to a mounting enthusiasm, of the same order as that of the child joyful in the discovery of his autonomy. Dance appears, therefore, as a privileged activity, one which reactivates the 'fort-da' which, as the inaugural game giving access to language and to the status of subject, is at the core of the therapeutic process. Thus we strive in Primitive Expression to reactivate its mechanism through the play of opposites. The reinforcing and re-actualising of the 'fort-da' take place via a diversity of different forms of this call–reply, involving not only movements, but also partners: reciprocal imitation, echoing alternation, gestural and musical games maintain a call–reply between group and group leader or between participants; or indeed between two different groups such as we find in choral dynamics. In the latter the group divides into subgroups who call and reply to each other, each one producing a gestural and vocal sequence in four time, echoed by a complementary sequence in the other group. Primitive Expression creates thereby a linkage, reproducing the 'fort-da' at the heart of the group.

'Calling' the Other/'Answering' himself

The novelty of the 'fort-da' consists in the capacity it awakens in the child to 'call' the absent one through the play of symmetrical opposites in the call–reply, superposed on the couple absence–presence and invisible–visible. The child is henceforth able to ground all the opposites experienced since birth (pleasure/displeasure, good breast/bad breast, inside/outside, mother/father, and so on) on the foundation of the opposition absence/presence. It attains thus the ability to use them as symbolic substitutes designating things in their absence: to evoke them, convoke them, in a 'call' which brings them 'magically' to presence.

Following, moreover, the recognition of absence as invisible presence, the call connects to the absent Other in a new way. It no longer simply precedes and calls for presence; it becomes concomitant with absence and names the other in its invisible existence. By 'calling' the other who has disappeared, we give it a name. The 'call' transforms, that is, into nomination, and as such takes on a double function: it both 'calls' to the other in the hope of rendering it present and visible, and designates this other in its absence. The name is at one and the same time call and symbolisation.

Dance, like children's games, proposes a dynamic, corporeal meditation on the linguistic foundations of the human being. While the founding acts outlined in this chapter may appear somewhat abstract and complicated to the reader, they constitute a familiar experience to the dancer because they animate the 'logic' of his body. The mechanism of the 'call' of the Other comes to life in the game of opposites where each movement 'calls' the Other, engendering as if automatically the presence of its opposite (Figure 10.2). It also comes to life, however, when the symbolic substitute (the gesture) is recognised as the visible reverse of the invisible absent which it calls.

Primitive dance also allows us to hear, therefore, the call of everything which exists to be symbolised: each gesture which disappears into absence, leaving the halo of a virtual and invisible presence, 'calls' the Other, its symmetrical opposite, to rise to presence on the 'other side' of the body: which is to say, to symbolise it through a new incarnation. In its self-effacement, movement engenders an invisible 'shadow' (in a descent to the underworld?). Now at the low point of its cycle, it calls to the absent double which is rising to presence on the other bank, which in turn evokes and 'calls' its partner. The visible being calls out to be symbolised, the invisible being calls to symbolise. We could express things a little differently: things search names, while names look for things to say.

Symbolisation emerges from the superposition of a series of oppositions: absence/presence, visible/invisible, the surface of things and the reality it conceals. The association of these couples transforms the symbolic substitute into the underside of the absent being, the reality which it 'calls' and which 'calls it'.

The 'speaking animal' is the one who calls to and represents the Other, ultimately to represent itself: the 'fort-da' is not only a consolation, but also a joyful event with therapeutic effects. The dance of fort-da in rhythm dance therapy will allow the patient to emerge as subject.

Representing oneself through the Other

The pair call–reply interchange in a circularity: the Other is represented by the gesture which 'calls' the dancer; the I by the gesture which 'replies' to the Other, in a 'reply' which also represents a 'call' to the Other, and so on.

The Other and the I call–reply to each other amorously from each side of the cleft which divides the subject, seeking to seduce each other. With each return of the gesture a new layer of meaning is added: the announced is beautiful and the announcing renders it all the more beautiful. Dance is an act of absolute love which leads the dancer to an exceeding of self in which he forgets himself and puts his disappointments, frustrations, wounds to one side for the sake of an anticipated image.

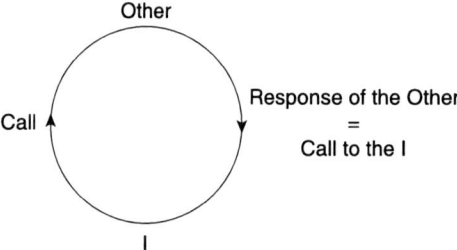

Figure 10.2 The circularity of the call–reply between I and the Other

The paternal function

The symbolisation requires the presence of a third person between mother and child, the 'father' (i.e. the paternal function which emerges with the presence of the 'Father' in the discourse of the mother). How are we to reconcile this idea with the transmission by the mother of the law through rhythmic practices: lullabies, imitative games, nursery rhymes, etc.?

Let us make first a sociological observation by remarking that the two roles are less carried out specifically by 'mother' and 'father' than by 'mama' and 'papa'.[1] Psychoanalysis conserves these evocative names to designate not people but two complementary functions: the first establishes the 'world of inside', the necessary love of self, the foundational narcissism of the infant, and the second leads the child to exit the maternal fold towards the 'outside world'. The two functions are today distributed indifferently between the two parents.

The same parent can fulfil both functions (e.g. single mothers) and from this perspective, the concept of the 'mother good enough' is particular interesting (Winnicott, 2005). This expression designates the mother as non-fusional, non-narcissistic, helping the baby to loosen its grip on her. Because she is not everything to her child, she leads it to invest in the outside and to love 'the father', which is to say the social, exterior world. Lacanian psychoanalysis calls it the paternal function or 'Le Nom du Père' and provides some interesting psychological and anthropological insights into the role of the 'fort-da' game.

The I and the Other call to each other in a reciprocal symbolisation through symbolic substitutes which the linguists name signifiers. The signifiers, which for Lacanian psychoanalysts are not only words, but also all kind of substitutes (e.g. drawings, gestures or sounds) symbolising each other by masking each other, in the same way that the Lascaux paintings superpose different animals: each one veils/unveils the one over which it is superposed, illustrating the mode of functioning of the symbolic chain. According to Lacan, 'language' (i.e. culture in general), makes up the 'treasure of signifiers' harvested by man from amidst all that which surrounds him (the Other) to spell out himself. For psychoanalysis, the signifiers without fail return ultimately to the subject via all the substitutes through which he represents the Other (i.e. himself).

By virtue of the reversible dialectic of the call–reply, the Other 'called' by man to signify him, 'responds' precisely by signifying him. Lacan summarises this process as follows: 'A signifier represents a subject for another signifier.' In effect, the signifiers do not refer directly back to the subject, because they signify through the signifiers of signifiers of, signifiers etc., up to the first signifier of the chain, etc., called by Lacan S1 or the phallic signifier, principal signifier which remains concealed, inaccessible to our consciousness. It is the inheritor of the archaic lived experience of the child, fashioned while the latter was a 'phallus' filling in the absence of its mother during the fusional stage prior to language. It sinks under the bar (veil) of 'repression' (i.e. primary repression) and belongs to the register of the Real.

The phallus, venerated in a number of societies via forms which evoke the penis, represents a vital force which must be 'civilised' to enable the passage from Nature to Culture (i.e. to give access to humanity). The ceremonies of the veiling/unveiling of the phallus are the key to the Greek Mysteries of Eleusis and the other mysteries of the ancient Mediterranean (Figure 10.3). Their most secret rite consists in unveiling a phallus before the initiated.

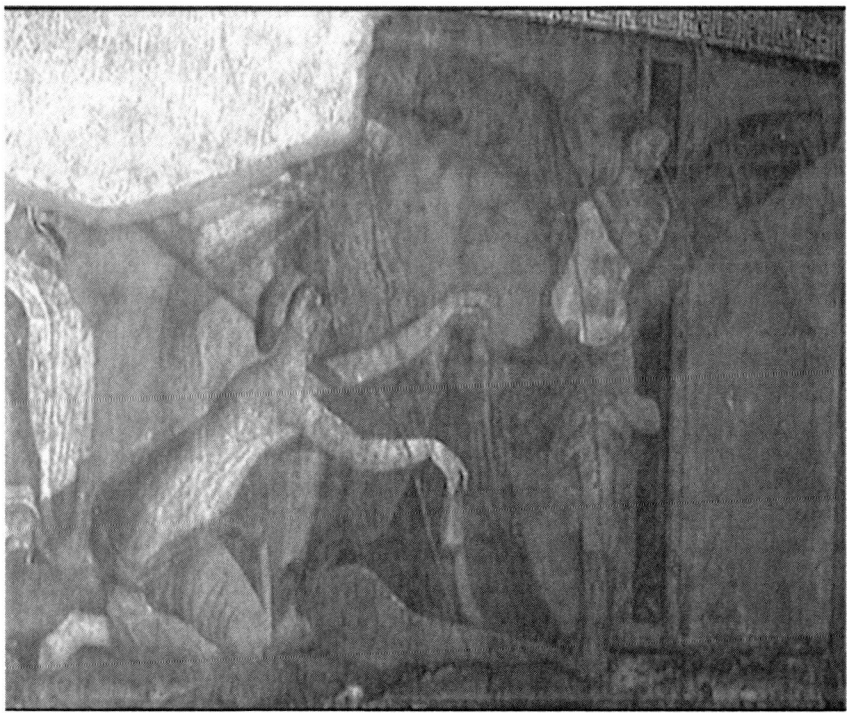

Figure 10.3 An initiated unveils the phallus, Villa of the Mysteries, 1st–2nd century BC, Pompeii

The idea of veiling corresponds exactly to that of repression in psychoanalysis. It presupposes that the child is willing to renounce fusion in a rupturing of the dyad which psychoanalysis calls 'castration'. The world of fusion passes under the 'bar' of repression and will no longer be accessible to consciousness. It will be forgotten and in its place stand symbolic substitutes which express it while travestying it, therefore 'veiling' it. The self-sacrifice of the child gives it access to language, in opposition to the silence of the *infans*, thus to humanity and culture, in opposition to animality and Nature.

We see that the signifier S1 has two faces: one is mute, turned towards the world of fusion (*jouissance*) and the unconscious; the other is of a linguistic nature, testifying to the renouncing of fusion and the separation which enables us to distinguish things by naming them. This psychic human reality is illustrated by the god Dionysius with his two faces, participating at the same time in savage Nature and Culture, permitting thereby the passage from one to the next.

The operation of 'castration' (i.e. cutting in the fusion, or veiling the phallus) is accomplished via the 'father' (i.e. the paternal function which can be worn also by the mother if she is 'good enough' but not 'too good' (i.e. fusional) who will lead the child to language by virtue of the discovery and use of paternal metaphor). To attain autonomy the child must renounce the carnal presence of the mother and replace her with a symbolic substitute, a process from which language emerges. Psychoanalysis gives the title 'paternal metaphor' to the primordial signifier which initiates the chain of the signifiers of signifiers of signifiers and so on. We will now look more closely at this stage, which is crucial to the therapeutic process.

It is, in fact, easy to understand. The child discovers that all departure is not death: the mother returns. The place where she goes when she leaves is not a place of destruction: it is not 'hell'. To the question 'but where does she go when she leaves?' the child finds a response: the outside, the 'father'. The child thereby associates two opposites: absence of the mother equals existence of the father. Through the game of 'fort-da', it 'calls' the mother through the 'name of the father'. The latter appears as the symbolic third on the basis of which the triangle father–mother–child is established, putting an end to symbiosis with the 'mother' (inside, imagination) which is a joyous yet deadening experience insofar as it leads to psychosis.

According to Lacan, the child has now gained the capacity to 'formulate absence'; to console himself with a symbolic substitute: 'the paternal metaphor' or 'name of the Father'. It will join from now on the absence of the mother to the presence of the father, ceasing to oppose the world of inside (the mother, imagination) to that of the outside (father) which he will use to symbolise the first. The child becomes capable of passing from the Imagination to the Symbolic, a path that every therapeutic process will have to retrace. Like the child, the patient must find the means to distance himself from the 'maternal' world of the inside, by associating her absence (which is to say the presence of the subject) to the paternal metaphor – a metaphor which designates ultimately the subject in the process of saying himself.

The psychotic was not forbidden the state of fusion and he remains in psychic symbiosis with the mother, a prisoner of the *jouissance* of the subject-object, of the state of fusion–confusion. According to the word play of Lacan, he does not have the 'Nom du Père'.

Lacan attributes to the founding operation of 'fort-da' the character of 'incantation', highlighting thus its 'sacred' character. Dance allows us to glimpse the climate of enthusiasm, therefore the relation to a transcendence which presides over the emergence of the subject, surging corporeally into being through the incarnated third term, the 'Nom du Père'. In the game of 'fort-da', it is the body which in binding the oppositions together rhythmically and naming thus the absence of the mother, also names the subject who appears when she disappears. The intoxication of dance seems to us to arise similarly from the surmounting of the division through the identification of the dancer to the rhythm which contains this division (through the absence which circulates between its two poles). Rhythm is the paradoxical object towards which the two opposed registers converge: fusion (the beating of the heart and maternal cradling); and separation (the 'Nom du Père'). The dancer dances with one foot in fusion, another in separation; with phallus both veiled and unveiled. He is the subject in its nascent state, identifying with the vital force at the point at which it becomes 'civilised', producing Culture while retaining all the power of Nature. Dance is one of the rare states in which these two aspects of human nature co-exist.

The paternal function in rhythm dance therapy

We understand that the recognition of the existence of the 'father' as object of the desire of the mother (responsible for her absences) is necessary to the constitution of the subject. We should not be surprised therefore that a great number of psychoses take place when the mother does not initiate the process of recognition of the father: when, for example, she 'erases' the father in her communication with the child. The child is thus bereft of the third pole which would allow it to exit fusion. The one who does not have the Other becomes psychotic.

In dance therapy we seek to create the third pole, that of the 'father', and through triangulation to associate it with the absence of the mother. We employ coupled gestures to direct their meaning to the couple Other-self and their reversed relation absence–presence. After all, the psychotic also engages in repetitive gestures, which prevents him from remaining in imaginary fusion to the mother. He comes and goes from one node to the other of the dyad, without ever exiting it.

He requires the 'third', whose existence dance therapy seeks to induce through a diversity of means. The patient must be led to understand that the therapist is himself subjected to an 'other' order, a law which exceeds him and prevents him from engulfing patients in his own desire. These are protected from fusion with him through the presence of 'safeguards' (e.g. rhythm, aesthetics, corporeal technique) and the framework of a respected tradition, which is to say, the movements form part of a pre-existing heritage which is in no way the product of his own fantasy.

Rhythm, often incarnated by the percussionist ('paternal' figure), is a key factor in dance therapy due to the role it plays in the materialisation of this third term (the 'father'), to which the mother (therapist) submits herself and which incites her to dance.

The case of Melanie, an adolescent referred to us by an institution for psychotic children, will help us to grasp this process. As an only and desired child, she grew up without any sign of difficulty until the age of 2. She was spoiled by her parents who loved her and each other. Then suddenly their world collapsed when her father died in a car accident. Disconsolate, the mother did not know how to reply to the questions of the child and hid the truth from her. For more than a year, she was told 'Daddy is going to return', that he was preoccupied by activities which she invented and recounted in detail. Thanks to her efforts, Melanie escaped sorrow; yet there are worse things than grief. Melanie began to become detached from the world and closed in on herself in an autistic withdrawal which soon required her hospitalisation. She began to speak to no one except her mother, and in a language so weakly articulated that they alone could understand each other.

When I met Melanie, she was 13, a pretty adolescent, slim, graceful and smiling. Yet whenever I attempted to speak to her, she would recoil in alarm and bury her face in her mother's shoulder. She explained that her daughter, despite a significant psycho-affective delay, had received some schooling in her institution. Over the last year, she had exhibited on numerous occasions a desire to dance, moving spontaneously on hearing certain musical rhythms. The institution, therefore, thought to place Melanie in our care.

I agreed with her mother that they would initially come to watch a session together. She would have preferred her daughter to have individual sessions in which she could take part, but I insisted on Melanie participating without her, my reasoning being that the adolescent should follow a collective activity rather than be in dual relation with the therapist in a situation resembling the state of fusion she experienced at home.

At the end of the observation session, mother and child agreed to start the following week. Her mother would bring Melanie to the session, before leaving us alone. She, in fact, experienced great difficulty in leaving Melanie. When they arrived, half an hour before the start of the session (in order to let the participants have a convivial exchange with each other or with the therapist and her assistant), they remained isolated together on a bench until the start of the exercises. Moreover, the mother always returned to pick up her daughter in advance, under a variety of pretexts (which I did not accept, finding it essential for Melanie to participate in the group until the end of the session).

From the first weeks the adolescent reacts as little to the rhythm as to the models proposed. Although she placed herself in front of the therapist, in the first row of participants, she never looked at her and her body seemed to float in space without attaching itself to the rhythm and entirely without grasping the gestures to be executed. Her corporeal range was very limited. She was incapable of bending her knees if we asked her, as she was of capturing the difference between the horizontality or verticality of the arms. She was indeed incapable of identifying the directions or even simply of orientating herself like the others so as to face the therapist. In effect, the body of Melanie never presented its frontal aspect: as furtive as her gaze, it escaped sideways in quarter or profile. During the set pieces in the room designed to bring participants into contact with each other, the adolescent circled like a shadow, without touching the others, though she did laugh and seemed to enjoy herself. Her mother confirmed to us that she very much enjoyed coming, which seemed to be a good omen, pleasure being essential to this form of therapy. Yet progress was slow. For the first few weeks, I rarely intervened and only ever to congratulate her when a sketchy movement indicated that she was present despite appearing to be 'elsewhere'.

Yet after three months her steps became more sure and anchored themselves to the ground. She followed the rhythm for more sustained periods and regained it whenever she lost it. Her grasp of time came much earlier than improvement in her sense of corporeal orientation, which did not really begin to improve until the fourth month. I noticed that her gaze, which was still incapable of fixing on the therapist, had nevertheless lost its wandering character to fix on a 'precise' object: the percussionist. This seemed to me to confirm that in the cure, the musician plays the role of the third, the separating agent who had begun to put to an end to the psychic fusion of Melanie with her mother (present in transferential terms in the person of the therapist) and to create a pole of exteriority by incarnating the Law of rhythm.

The separation of the two parties of the dyad mother–child had not taken effect for Melanie, less because of the real absence of the dead father, than because of the inability of her mother to articulate this death, to speak of it (symbolise this absence): to say goodbye to her husband, exit her depression and invest in any object other than her daughter.[2] Melanie remained engulfed in that fusion.

The percussionist played in this case the role of the father, not only because he presented a masculine figure, but also because he allowed the adolescent to understand that the rhythm that she incarnated ruled equally the steps and movements of the therapist. The transferential 'mother' did not obey her own 'caprices' but submitted herself to the rule of the rhythm reigning over the entire group.

Having perceived and recognised this 'paternal' existence, Melanie began to respond to the rhythm and to base her movement on it. At the end of eight months of therapeutic work, she was capable of imitation, of organising her corporeal schema and of communicating with the other dancers. She also stopped placing herself in the front row and began to place herself behind a participant, Michel, to whom she addressed wide smiles and whose gestures she reproduced (including the errors). She opened herself, affirmed herself, communicated and made, according to her educators, significant progress at school. She remained, however, bereft of speech; until one day, at the start of the session, she suddenly and entirely naturally enquired about two participants who held particular meaning for her: 'Are Michel and Roger going to come this evening?'

By virtue of the discovery of the third which had rendered her able to grasp the 'fort-da' and the paternal metaphor, Melanie had attained both the autonomy of separation (evinced by the improvement in the assuredness of her bearing, manifesting an awareness of her body as a distinct entity) and language.

If, unfortunately budgetary constraints rarely allow the use of a percussionist, the dance therapist must clearly allocate the role of the third to rhythm even if materialised through a simple recording. The drum is the universal instrument of shamanism and an essential tool in traditional dance therapy. We, in turn, accord it its full importance in Primitive Expression because the rhythm is the basis of the 'fort-da' which, following Lacan, is a kind of trance, an incantation to the Other, a mystical experience. By seeking through rhythm a reactivation of the call–reply with the Other, the dancer feels that something 'dances' in his body drawing towards the trance of rhythm.

A de-centred ego

Trance is the experience of absence–presence: the interchangeability of the poles call–reply leads one to celebrate an ideal Other which incarnates itself in the dancer sometimes to the point of confusion (possession) (Figure 10.4). The mystics see in absence the face of God: the absolute, the totally Other, so it is not surprising that they approach its essence through corporeal rhythmic techniques (Indian *mantras*, sufi *dikr*, etc.). Dance clearly demonstrates the fashion in which the call–reply initiates the amorous quest for the Other in the identification with absence. The circularity of the repetitive gesture renders the call of the dancer to the Other, which is identical to the response of the Other to the dancer. This reversibility, in turn, results in an interchangeability – an identity between the dancer and the Other – which justifies the etymology of the word enthusiasm ('to have a god in oneself') applied to the state of trance (ecstasy or possession).

Dance is, therefore, at its deepest roots, a mystical technique to the extent that the dyad dancer/Other risks collapsing in much the same fashion as the dyad man/God for the mystics. In both cases the end result is the celebration of the Other in place of the ego. This should lead to a reconsideration of the famous

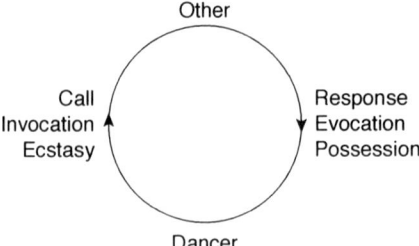

Figure 10.4 Circularity of call–reply between the dancer and the Other

'narcissism' of dance. That the ego becomes the Other does not mean that it is 'divinised'. In dance it is not the dancer who is venerated, but the Other as a figure proposed to the ego as its Ideal, one which it attempts to incarnate in the dancing body.

It is a question, therefore, not of a paranoid confusion in which the dancer of the mystic 'would take himself' for God, but tries to know him (and therefore himself) through a mystical experience of an absence. Angelus Silesius describes it thus: 'We do not know what God is. He is neither light nor spirit. He is what neither you nor I nor any creature can feel except by becoming what He is' (Silesius, 1983: 31).

Individuation

Individuation is a therapeutic effect of symbolisation, rendering possible the attachment to that which is missing (the absent object) to a representation. The child initially will hallucinate this object if it does not have it. For example, when the mother is distant, the infant 'hallucinates' the breast, which temporarily procures the same satisfaction as the real breast. Later, he will represent it through the image of the breast itself, then through substitutes. The object of the oral drive (the breast) can accordingly be represented alternatively by the dummy, bottle, parts of the mother's body which the child touches while suckling, clothes carried by her during a moment of satisfaction and well-being or, on the contrary, during the course of a traumatising experience of hunger and frustration. The child 'will choose', amongst the infinity of possible signifiers which the surrounding world offers. He will attach his drive to representations of situations and the affective states linked to these situations by virtue of the way others acted within them and responded to him personally. Given that each human story is different, each individual carries his own representations and there are no two individuals who possess the same cluster of representations. Symbolising his drives corresponds, therefore, to investing his own particular representations in them (which engenders in each person particular modes of behaviour), constructing thereby his own singular (ideal) identity.

As we have seen, symbolising the missing object (e.g. the mother) ultimately corresponds to symbolising oneself (ideal, other) for the child. We saw that once Melanie could use rhythm to represent the third which would separate her from her mother, she was also able to symbolise all kinds of drive elements with her body. Before she started to speak, she had begun to 'live' her movements – to feel herself separated enough from her mother's body to invest them with meaning. This is a very important dimension of dance therapy. According to the way in which participants reproduce the gestures transmitted to them by the therapist, we can measure the extent to which these gestures have acquired the capacity to represent them. If they are executed in a mechanical way, without 'soul', the individual cannot use them to symbolise himself. He does not recognise himself in them, which might occur even to dancers with good technique. However, a movement which is 'branched into' the affective dimension, and capable, thereby, of serving as the bearer of the corresponding drive, can immediately be recognised. We call this a 'lived' movement.

Notes

1 Let us not forget that the notion of the 'father' in Lacanian psychoanalysis can be understood in terms of the 'outside', the Other. They are therefore 'names of the outside', or otherwise put, the words of language (and not the name of the 'papa' which will come to symbolise the mother, by virtue of the associations the child will attach to it).
2 To be understood in the psychoanalytical sense of the word (e.g. as an 'object of love').

Part IV
The therapeutic process

11 The healing process

According to psychoanalytical theory, therapy does not only consist in pacifying the drives, it is also involves symbolic reorganisation. This means that the drives must link to representations other than those which led to the pathology, which arises from a fault in symbolisation: either the drive is not symbolised and 'errs' in the organism by awakening anxiety, or it is represented by a pathogenic symbolisation which is destructive or devalourising. For example, if the drive is represented by figures such as monsters or wolves, the child will be subject to anxieties of destruction and of being devoured which could, if they are excessive, make it regress to a stage where it lives its body as dismembered. It is, therefore, essential in therapy, to endow the subject with the capacity of linking its drives to other representations: either those which the therapist proposes from the exterior, as we saw in the case of the shaman, or those which the subject produces himself, which is the case in the psychoanalytical cure.

In both cases, symbolic representation organises the drive by 'containing' it, channelling its flux through the mould of the signifier. The symbol functions, therefore, as a trigger for the energy of the drives, but also as a regulator which organises its course.

If symbolisation consists in representing the object of the drive (or in other words lack, therefore, of desire, which is to say the self) through substitutes, it is faced with an infinite task: the diversity of objects to be named is enormous (since the drives are multiple) as are the number of signifiers which represent them and designate the subject through symbolic representations (verbal or non-verbal).

The creation of meaning

The symbols, however arbitrary they appear, insofar as they no longer attempt to imitate, appear as 'more true' than the visible thing because they give access, beyond the exterior aspect, to its very essence. This recalibration of the relation to the world corresponds to the creation of a meaning which goes beyond the exterior aspect of the object. For this reason, Winnicott calls it the 'object found-created'. It is fundamental to art therapy, as there is no therapy without the creation of meaning.

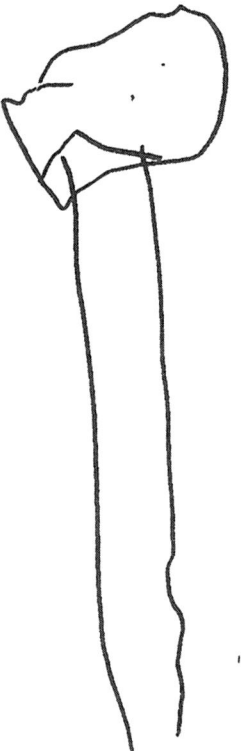

Figure 11.1 Drawing of a tadpole man by a 4-year-old child

To take an example, a teacher took her pupils outside to draw, seating them next to a viaduct. After one hour, she collected their drawings. One struck her in particular: one child had drawn boots in the form of the arches of the viaduct. The child was Paul Klee. However, all children possess this capacity to recreate the world and to see the viaducts walking.

The particular character of the human psyche is tied to this welcoming of the exterior symbol as a call to grasp the essence of the thing: an essence which the human being distils from appearance (since it exists even in absence), in intimate relation with his own individual essence destined for death and separation. The symbol reveals to it in an illumination that things survive death, have a 'beyond', a 'soul' which speaks to him of his own soul (Figure 11.1).[1]

This is perhaps the reason why the child engages with the objects of the world in a dialogue of such intensity. Everything speaks to it, becomes symbolic: all things represent something else, ultimately the child itself, in a game of infinite reflections. Meaning is from now on to be found everywhere. It permeates the young human, embodying a centripetal dynamic by speaking 'to it' and a centrifugal dynamic by speaking 'of it'.

In the realm of art therapy, which is of the character of a transitional activity, those forms participate at the same time in the simulacra and the 'non-resembling' sign (e.g. the tam-tam as a musical evocation of the beating of the heart). It may also take its distance from them, sometimes to the point of abstraction. In the 'primitive' arts, representation situates itself between similarity and arbitrariness by appealing to stylisation and the simplification of forms (Schott-Billmann, 2001: 119). These are orientated towards the essence of things rather than their appearance. This renders them capable of reactivating the joy felt by the child upon the realisation of its ability to represent (the Symbolic) in the surging to presence of the model according to the logic of the structure rather than formal resemblance. The setting up of this difference demonstrates the child's ability to take absence into account, allowing him to escape from the 'prison' of appearance to (re)create reality.

An example will show the importance of this 'revelation' via artistic form within the framework of child therapy. Marcel, aged 5, was 'polite but a dreamer at school' and a bed wetter. He appeared to have to forgotten about the existence of his father, indeed his very name, who had left three years previously and who had been rapidly 'replaced' by his mother's new companion. His mother indeed had actively tried to erase the memory of this bearded and coarse figure who had been the source of much worry for her. She never spoke to her child of Grégoire, his biological father. His photo remained, among others, by the front door, yet it raised no questions or comments, no more on the part of the mother than of Marcel (who would pass by his father's photo without appearing to notice it). Yet one day, in a therapy session 'in front of the mirror', the child began to paint his face like a clown. He tried one design, which he abandoned, then started a second in which he suppressed only the eyebrows so as to realign them. He added 'to make it pretty', some cross-hatchings of black crayon on the chin. He looked at himself fixedly and said in a dreamy voice as if from afar, 'it looks like Grégoire'. The latter had appeared as a revelation, by the suggestion of the stylised beard; the distance which stylisation affords had encouraged this insight.

This stage, which the animal never attains, corresponds to the overcoming of the decoy, replacing it with substitutes in the form of representations which do not imitate, but rather signify. Yet, we have seen that in symbolisation, the human being also represents himself. This is the source of its difference from imitation. The symbol can be found in all human productions: music which makes use of sounds, dance which makes use of rhythmic movement, and of course verbal language which uses acoustic forms. These different modes of expression link us to the world because, through the symbols which represent them, all things have a double: the entire world, including our imagination, can exist in symbolic fashion.

Words look for things to 'say', things words to 'say' them. Similarly, on the one hand, the forms, whether abstract or imitative, look for things to represent, either by signifying them through the symbol or by duplicating them through the image. On the other hand, things, those of the exterior world but equally of the psychic universe, 'call' the human being to take up this work. Delivered to themselves, forms and things cannot meet. It is, therefore, the task of the individual to respond to this double call by binding things and their representation whether in pictorial form (appearance) or symbolic form (essence).

Like the child of the Gardners, we rejoice when we reunite forms with their things, all the more so when in these forms sign and image converge (absence and presence, structure and appearance, soul and body, life and death), and even more still when this operation involves the body as in dance.

The therapeutic character of arts therapy is particular to it; it is neither that of psychoanalysis nor emotional therapies, which have no ambition towards artistic expression. Its nearest cousin is the shamanic cure. Like the shaman, art therapy brings together the role of therapist and artist, curing through the mechanism of symbolic effectiveness.

Symbolic reorganisation

Symbolisation in artistic, plastic, musical, gestural and verbal forms constitutes an essential dimension of art therapy. Such forms function, in effect, as substitutes serving to represent the drives and therefore the subject. Artistic productions, wherever received or emitted, connect representations to the body. Let us remember that the coding of drives in symbolic forms which contain them and represent them in a way which is acceptable to the super-ego (and which are capable of carrying meaning for the subject, as we will see in Chapter 12) is at the foundation of the psychic reorganisation on which therapy sets its sights.

Let us take an example: a clinical case reported by Jean-Yves Collart, a dance therapist at the hospital of Havre. It concerns a 16-year-old girl whom we will call Sarah.[2]

Sarah

She arrived at the workshop for the first time accompanied by a nurse who did not remain during the session. Sarah was an adolescent adorned with make-up which appeared to have been put on very hastily, and which in no way corresponded to the form of her face. Her movements obeyed a similar logic: she moved forward with a rapid and disarticulated step to such an extent that she appeared to run the constant risk of spraining her ankle.

It was also clear that each singular movement was not in synchrony with the ensemble of her body, giving the impression, through the delay between each partial movement, that each joint moved completely independent of the body. It seemed indeed that she exaggerated each movement in order to overcompensate for this delay, so that each time it was as if she was attempting to avoid an imminent fall. I saw in the drama expressed by her physical gait a significant physical dismembering at work.

In addition, Sarah was incapable of remaining still. Her dyskinesias were perhaps secondary to neuroleptic treatment; however, this did not present akathisia. Rather she gave the impression of collapsing on a chair or couch in leaning to the right or left in exaggerated fashion. In her movement Sarah evoked to me something of the invertebrate in search of a vertebral column. For this reason, although she had been referred to me for a session of active music therapy, I preferred to orientate rapidly the sessions towards a programme centred on rhythmic dance therapy: Primitive Expression.

Sarah had a low level of educational attainment, was culturally poor and had a very difficult family background which had led her to be placed in a foster family. Bursts of violent behaviour had subsequently resulted in full-time hospitalisation in a psychiatric ward.

The first session was cut short because Sarah sat at my side and addressed me in familiar terms (a common practice within the institution, yet which I do not accept in the interest of the patient towards whom it is necessary to establish distance). She pretended to lift her skirt, and then attempted to hit me on the arms several times. I indicated my desire to be addressed more formally, and subsequently stressed the necessity of organising the sessions otherwise. Thus, in collaboration with her reference team, we planned sessions with an accompanying artist who would actively participate.

The triadic situation (with the accompanying artist) was felt as less dangerous than a dual relation (with me), and Sarah was, in the following sessions, able to listen to advice and engage with the course of therapy more serenely.

The ritualising of the sessions allowed us to define their progression to a high degree of precision.

We started by singing the first name of each individual in the triad with the assistance of a xylophone through which we produced a binary rhythm accompanying a binary gestural movement. Sometimes we would take turns, sometimes we would act together. Cultivating this perspective of group work, presented as a ritual of entry, encouraged Sarah first of all to respect a binary rhythmic law given by herself, following the model of a group which respects this same law. In addition, the improvisation of first names to a rhythm raised to the status of law enabled Sarah in my opinion to envisage relationships in other terms than those of the pseudo-eroticising and violent attitudes to which she had been the plaything perhaps since her early childhood.

I then proposed a dance to a binary rhythm produced by a recording of the djembé. The choreography of the dance was based on two axes (forwards/backwards), then on four axes (forwards/backwards/left/right). Following together the rhythm of the djembé, we made four steps forwards and four steps backwards during which Sarah decided, with my support, to imitate a lion. I suggested two aspects of the lion to her, ferocious and gentle. We danced the first four beats in advancing step, performing a ferocious lion which made use of its aggression to catch its prey. For the four following beats, performed while moving backwards, we transformed ourselves both into a cat and the human who strokes it while chanting 'meow'.

My partner was not at all at ease with this type of exercise, which appeared too childish for her. Sarah, however, burst out laughing at each pause, asking us to repeat the exercise, introducing indeed with each repetition more intentionality into her movements. Quite remarkably, she began to lose her dyskinesias during the moments of rest between repetitions.

This exercise allowed Sarah to act out through play, and in a way which was adapted to infantile psychosis, two extreme attitudes which had manifestly throughout the course of her life determined her way of relating to the world. It was perhaps for her the opportunity to come to terms with the violence she had experienced by addressing it through the prism of a body submitting itself to the law of rhythm, a law which is not without relation to the fundamental law which allows us to become social animals. She was, perhaps, in turn, able to revisit the seduction of the child who desires to be hugged by acting out the person who strokes the cat, while at the same time taking her distance from the more adult and ambivalent seduction she had experienced during the course of her childhood.

These are evidently only hypotheses and would require more investigation to substantiate. What was in any case clear is that this little exercise helped Sarah to acquire a more sure and harmonious posture.

This was true to such an extent that our sessions concluded with a competitive and playful exercise in which the goal was to hold a little bamboo stick on the head as long as possible by alternating set postures and effecting a promenade across the length of the room.

Symbolisation proposed within a rhythmic and strongly ritualised framework had allowed us to recognise, contain and express the ambivalence of Sarah, an ambivalence which is particularly strong in the psychotic subject, yet which exists in all human beings and must be addressed by each one of us symbolically.

Pacifying, mastering and structuring

In rhythm dance therapy, Primitive Expression involves a mastering of the body insofar as it implies production (vocal and gestural) accomplished through the intermediary of the musculature. It thus appeases the anxiety which may, in some cases, submerge the subject and which always risks resurging (e.g. anxiety of a phobic character, anxiety of castration and its secondary forms: the anxiety of separation and of death, anxiety of the unknown, and so on). It offers us, alongside the pleasure taken in the mastery of the body, the opportunity to experiment with and give our approval to the erogenous pleasure of a body whose movement is contained and channelled by structured yet nevertheless intensely active (particularly in dance when at the maximum of its effort, vivacity and desire).

Finally, it renders possible an interweaving of desire and law by posing limits and rules. These may engender suffering and confront the subject with interdiction (in dance, for example, where it is forbidden to pass to the act itself); yet ultimately the pacifying of the anxiety engendered by transgression allows us to understand the sense of security which the limits put in place by the Law provides. The success of the 'works' created 'according to the rules of art' can only produce positive, structuring effects on the one who has accepted its framework and integrated it into the productions through which he affirms himself and proves his own existence.

It is of secondary concern whether art therapy leads the patient to incorporate external symbolic forms as in the case of the shaman, or whether these forms involve improvisations: what ultimately counts is that dance therapy leads the subject to invest meaning in the signifiers which permeate him, which speak to him and speak of him; that he appropriates them in order to represent himself. He symbolises, thus, his existence in the world, indeed creates himself, by weaving self and world together, setting in motion a poetic call–reply between its forms and his self-understanding. The metamorphoses rendered possible by dance therapy are therefore the result of symbolic efficacy.

We should add that art therapy is not only a technique, but also a relation between patient and therapist in which a transfer takes place through artistic language. The therapist must also be 'recognised' by the patient, who cannot become autonomous and emerge as 'I' so long as he does not feel the existence of the 'other'.

Sublimation

The origins of sublimation are to be found in the body since it is instinctual energy which triggers and fuels its mechanism, defined by Freud as the deflection of drives towards 'more noble and social valuable' goals without offering any further explanation. If we concur with Freud that there are three great sublimations – science, religion and art – we notice that they all seek to explore domains which exceed the register of human existence: the first strives to uncover the mysteries behind the functioning of nature, the second attempts to approach the divine, the third to create 'another' world beyond appearance in which the essence of things is revealed. They constitute three different paths towards the interrogation of the invisible.

When engaging with art we must understand it both in terms of its traditional mould as the search for beauty, as well as its rethinking from Marcel Duchamp onwards. The therapeutic value of this vision of art, distorted within certain types of dance via banalisation and self-exhibition, remains to be shown. We thus prefer to analyse a mechanism which has already largely proved its value: sublimation as the search for a going beyond all limits, not in the provocation and display of the self; rather in the search for an 'elevation' towards a domain which no longer speaks of the self but of the universal. In our pursuit of this mechanism, we will once more follow the path of the child.

Sublimation, even if it traces its course within the symbolic dimension, does not rest content with it. It unveils the aspiration of man to exceed its own ego towards an ideal ego. The latter is not without relation to the former, though this would be an ego transcended in the encounter with the Other: it is of the order of mystical experience. Sublimation aims to incarnate the beauty encountered on the banks of the sacred. It is the noble activity of humanity, the quest for the essence of the world which surrounds it: the mystery of being-in-the-world, the essence of God, the nature of the Other constitutes the heart of the enigma with which humanity has grappled for millions of years.[3] It is already present in the games of the child who questions the world in an intense dialogue which he carries out with things. The arrival of adulthood, however, can discourage him in his quest; he often reduces the object to its function. For most 'big people', a chair is only a chair, a vase is only a vase, whereas the child interrogates the chair or vase from all possible angles.

Sublimation involves the transformation of love for the world into mystical love for its hidden face, which alone reveals what He is. The second partner, the human, engages him in an amorous call–reply which involves both speaking and listening, creation and meditation. Indeed creation emerges from an act of mystical love between man and the soul of the world (Other). It is as such that the individual speaks the Other and hears It; that the Other can be unveiled through the human individual, who is alone in being able to register its response. It is in this sense that, in similar fashion to the child who by naming his mother defines himself, the adult comes to his own identity by striving to decipher the enigma of the Other. The difference in the experience of sublimation lies in the fact that it allows the adult to express what is most beautiful within himself, in his aspiration to exceed all limits, to attain an ideal through which he will gain access to the 'sublime'. Just as the child recognises himself in anticipatory fashion in the image of the mirror before he is able to represent himself through it, we allow ourselves to hope that sublimation, by proposing figures of the Other through which man gives the best of himself, harbours the promise of what the future holds. Insofar as it addresses an ego ideal, sublimation implicitly considers man as perfectible. It may as such represent a vehicle for progress, perhaps indeed the most 'noble' human activity since it both announces and impels us to move towards a future humanity.

Primitive aesthetics

Dance therapy involves both symbolisation (saying something with the body) and, when the patient is capable of it, sublimation (expressing oneself through exceeding oneself in the beauty of the gesture). The primitivist aesthetic of the 'primitive' dance is not that of classical dance, which is not the same as contemporary dance, itself different from folk or tribal dance. Each choreographic production has its own style and unique beauty. The 'primitivist' aesthetic of Primitive Expression forms part of the contemporary current (Goldwater, 1966; Rubin, 1984) which appeals to tribal dances in a search, informed by contemporary western sensibilities, for stylisation, sobriety, the purity of the line (Figure 11.2). It supposes, therefore, on the part of the dancer a certain degree of 'sacrifice': a renouncing of the 'baroque' exuberance of movement for the simplicity of the line; a stripping away of certain elements considered to be gracious in other techniques, the curving of the fingers in classical dance or the fluidity of the *port de bras* in contemporary dance. There is an eschewing of the narcissistic satisfaction in 'prettifying' or in manifestations of seduction such as the swaying of the hips prevalent in a number of dances. We must allow the 'being of the gesture' to unfold, which is to say reveal its structure glimpsed/veiled under the movement

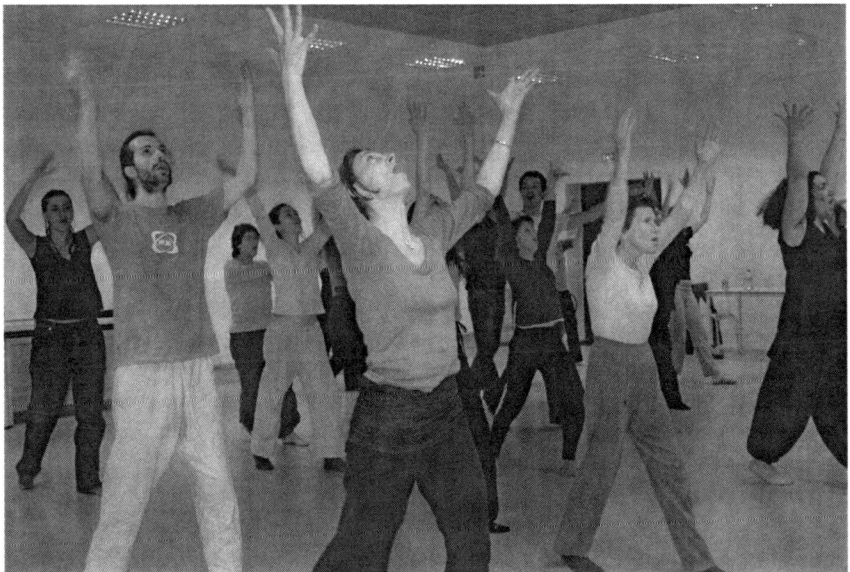

Figure 11.2 Primitive aesthetics: force and stylisation
Source: Photo by Caroline Schott

proposed. The outline of the essence becomes progressively sharper to the extent that the dancer, who works to inhabit the gesture, gives himself over to its inner form. This process requires deconstruction: a purification of the parasitic or inhibitive elements clouding our perception of this form.

The 'essence' of gesture unveils itself little by little to the dancer like a sacred alphabet progressively discovered (created) by his body. This essence implants itself in the human individual as soon as this individual 'concerns himself' with it and can invest in it, which is to say, give it a symbolic value manifested by the expressive character of the gesture. While each gesture resonates differently in the body of the dancer, it is nonetheless easy to discern in the intensity emanating from his movement if the Other has taken root.

'Primitive' dances, in binding the I and Other, lead the dancer to celebrate the Other through the ego ideal which results from their interaction. They allow us to see the purity of the essence of the Absence unique to the Other. The abandoning of ornamentation or details, in the tracing of a force which permeates and stretches out the body in a stylisation of lines, goes hand-in-hand with a stripping of the ego down to its essentials in the quest for transcendence. The 'primitivist' aesthetic seeks the Other and Primitive Expression is a dance of the Other, even if it is to the individual ego that it attaches itself, a fact which gives to each dancer his 'signature' and unique style .

Abandoning the narcissistic illusion of being all powerful, the dancer often feels himself 'purified' after a session. This seems to me to originate not only in the catharsis (purification, in Greek) obtained through the discharge of affects through the actions proposed, but also in the effect of purification of the movement itself. In this requirement of 'purity', in other words there is castration: which is say, a renouncing of the narcissistic feeling of being all powerful out of respect to the Other who is not the self, yet whose beauty the self tries to incarnate by purifying his gestures. By endowing the movement which represents the Other with the greatest possible accuracy, truth and authenticity, stripped of any element of flattery or seduction, the dancer attains sublimation. This involves the incarnation of the ego ideal as a figure of the Other, a powerful therapeutic factor.

This position of de-centring, which allows us to glimpse the ideal Other at the core of human existence, leading the latter to exceed itself in an ascending dynamic, corresponds closely to the spirit of modern thought: psychoanalysis sustains the movement initiated by Galileo and continued by Darwin who, from within their respective disciplines (astronomy and natural sciences), led us to see that man is no longer the centre of the world. Did Freud not return incessantly to the fashion in which the mastering ego finds itself 'put in its place' by the discovery of the unconscious which governs us without our knowledge and submits us to the unknown by escaping the control of 'clear reason'? The 'primitive dances' are close to this 'new' vision of things since they bring us to the realisation that it is through the body (and not in the separation of the body and soul) that the binding of the I to the Other is accomplished.[4] In primitive dance, the subject experiences what it is like to be permeated by the Other in its subjection to the rhythm which, working in parallel with the repetition of the gesture, guides trance towards this binding.

Primitive Expression is not based on dualism; it is a vital testament to the truth that will, reason, emotion and soul are as much corporeal as spiritual. This holistic vision resonates with the recalibrated sensibility of the twentieth and twenty-first centuries which challenges dualism and apprehends the human being in terms which are closer to those employed by shamanic societies. What is new in the confrontation with 'primitive' cultures is not the exoticism of their pagan rites but, on the contrary, their strange familiarity and profound fraternity with our current sensibilities.

The contemporary character of tribal dances explains why the choreographers of today are more interested than ever in primitive elements and draw on the immense reservoir of traditional dances. While such choreographers do not always refer to them explicitly, Primitive Expression is inspired overtly by these dances, so rich and yet so summarily treated by classical ethnology. It wishes to aid the West to invest corporeally in the quest for its symbolic, mythological wellspring on the basis of an enquiry into our origins. This is a quest which leads man to the recognition that he exists only in relation to the world, a relation in which, as the phenomenologist philosophers underline it, the body plays an essential role. 'The body is the vehicle for "being in the world", as Heidegger (Heidegger, 2009: 259) or Merleau–Ponty remind us.

From a scientific perspective, the individual researcher detaches himself from his subjectivity to attain complete objectivity (i.e. he separates himself from his object of study). In the mystical quest, however, as we have seen, the subject unites itself with his object while paradoxically remaining conscious of separation. The dancer occupies two positions simultaneously; he is both subject and object: the one who dances and the one who 'is danced'; the one who controls his movement and the one who is carried away or 'transported' by the Other. Such is the experience of Primitive Expression which presents itself as a 'moderated trance' permitting the dancer to corporeally interrogate his origins in an unmanning which reactivates them almost unwittingly. He thus awakens the joyful feeling of the non-narcissistic relation to the Other which rhythm, repetition, harmonics, symmetry and opposition render possible.

He 'encounters himself' in this new representation which is comforting, positive, valorising and which refers not only to what he is at this present moment, but what he will become. This hope invested in the future leads to a reorientation of his self-image and as such is conducive to the process of 'healing'.

We will give two examples of dance therapy in which sublimation played an essential role.

Laurette: reconstruction of the image of the body

Laurette, who was 22, arrived at my workshop. Her hand had been crushed in a car accident which had taken place ten months before the beginning of therapy. After a series of delicate operations, the surgeons had been able to restore a degree of functionality to two fingers, though the rest remained unsightly.

She was referred to us by her psychotherapist whom she had been meeting regularly 'following a bout of a depression following the accident', though she formulated her request to me exclusively in orthopaedic terms concerning the re-education of the hand.

With Laurette, however, the narcissistic wound concerned her entire body which she hid under drab clothes. She was inhibited, timid and her artificial smile was the only 'make-up' which she allowed herself. Her forced smile manifestly concealed a profound despair. Laurette felt herself to be not just ugly: she believed herself repulsive, monstrous, horrible to behold, as if she had entirely become her ruined hand, as if she were no longer anything but it.

Putting her in a situation in which she would need straightaway to confront the gaze of other participants was evidently out of the question. She would first require individual sessions. She would first of all need to escape from the cycle of self-negation. This did not involve ignoring the stump, rather putting it in its proper place as a part of the body: as unpleasant certainly, yet not as constitutive of the entirety of the physical or psychic reality of the young girl. Little by little, she accepted the idea that, even if dance could improve the performance of her hand, she had first to reconcile herself with her body image literally invaded by negativity, as if the hand represented to the eyes of the world what it represented to her: an object of horror.

During the first few weeks, she was incapable of investing in the gestures. Her attitude amounted to a kind of 'sabotage' designed to scupper in the most non-aesthetic fashion their performance. This made her even more ugly in her eyes, though her goal was to disappoint and disgust the therapist. Laurette bore within herself, and thus upon herself and also upon others, a malevolent and hateful gaze which dated from long before the accident, itself to a large extent brought about by her desire for self-destruction. It, without doubt, had its origin in the gaze of her mother, though of course there was no verbalisation during our sessions; which did not mean that there was no transfer, face to face with the therapist, of the admiring ambivalence (i.e. jealousy) that she had felt in the past towards her mother.

The bearing of the therapist, her understanding, benevolent and positive attitude are evidently of key importance in this type of cure. It was necessary to accept the death drives of Laurette in her seeking to destroy the therapeutic labour by systematically spoiling the movements which could have rendered her beautiful and gratified the therapist. Yet over time, the repetition of movements, the vehicle of a powerful affirmation of life, called to Laurette, almost unknown to her, awakening the desire to lead the gesture towards a more gratifying execution. This improvement induced a lowering of the vigilance of the superego which, satisfied by the effort made to render the gesture beautiful, showed itself to be less persecutory, and gradually the movements of Laurette took on the aspect of a young girl assured of herself. Her gestural production became more fluid, more harmonious. She indeed began to express herself with a certain tenderness, as if she were addressing her movements to someone whom she wanted to please. We chose this moment to introduce a video session. Laurette expressed her satisfaction with the image of herself which the recording presented, one which neither avoided nor searched out her hand. After 14 months in individual sessions held once a week, we decided to start her on group sessions.

The positive development continued. Laurette decided herself to participate in weekend sessions which, unlike weekly group sessions, involved recording and improvisation. From the start she was at ease with seeing herself on screen, an experience to which she had already been introduced in individual sessions. Yet the improvisations remained a source of anxiety to her, which was entirely understandable: she did not want to expose herself to the gaze of the others in situations where the one who improvises is the focal point of the group assembled around her without the protection of the 'gestural veil' of a coded movement. Arriving at this point in her journey, Laurette was not the only one to refuse such a risk: her problem, in other words, had become ordinary.

Three years after her first session of Primitive Expression, Laurette was able to improvise during sessions. She indeed appeared so natural in this exercise that, as a discussion group with a few participants would later show, most present had not even noticed her damaged hand.

Jacques and the deculpabilising of pleasure

Jacques was a scientist, and a classic case of obsessive-compulsive disorder. His rigour and methodical spirit had brought him success in the domain of research; yet an ensemble of constricting personal rituals, along with serious hypochondriac preoccupations and a relational difficulty with other researchers in his team, had brought him to psychoanalysis. This proved rapidly to be a disappointment due to Jacque's inability to allow himself to let go sufficiently to follow the association of his ideas. One person in his laboratory had spoken to him about Primitive Expression. Yet when he presented himself to me, he did not declare any explicit therapeutic need, simply the desire to relax after work. He attended weekly sessions, therefore, as he would a sport.

From the start, Jacques showed good coordination and a satisfying consciousness of his body. He displayed difficulties with rhythm – often encountered in those who strive to control themselves and who are not able to let go. This fear of letting go manifested itself in weak, inhibited movements. He resisted any extension of the body and could not hold his arms vertically, projecting perhaps onto the therapist a castration anxiety, preferring to remain huddled up before the menace. During the improvisation stage proposed at the end of each session, he confined himself to a poor and stereotyped performance.

Yet, as with Laurette, the process took effect little by little and almost unbeknown to him, short-circuiting, in some measure, his resistance. His movements became more expansive and his anxiety decreased. Repetition was reassuring for him as the gestures executed had not resulted in catastrophe. He could thus repeat them while risking venturing a little further, becoming a little more assertive. His transferential relationship improved; his movements became more confident: more risky and less 'miserly'. One of his greatest difficulties was taking pleasure in gestural production. For one month, Jacques limited himself to mechanical execution, a lifeless reproduction of the model, a sort of gymnastics deprived of signification and emotional investment. If he felt joy, he concealed it carefully under the obligation to follow instructions correctly, or in the satisfaction of accomplishing a procedure, the acquisition of knowledge: the 'knowing how to dance' that he could add to his panoply of scholarly achievements.

In a case like this we must be patient, and wait for the lure of life to manifest itself on the day when the superego, sufficiently pacified by the requirement for correct movement, leaves a little room for desire. It was necessary to show the patient the possibility of an authentic expression of himself which was not threatening, while authorising and encouraging him discreetly to continue to reassure the superego by insisting on respect for the rules.

In the case of obsessive neurosis, the execution of symbolisation through the coded gesture is essential. Desire must always be expressed within the Law, which is the only means of protecting the subject from the vengeance of a superego rendered dangerously unsatisfied by the arrival of pleasure without any measure of its opposite.

Respect for the superego's defences is a pre-condition for the success of the cure. Here, we demanded that Jacques not only correctly reproduced the proposed gestures, but also with an aesthetic perfection. It was on these terms that he accepted to make 'feminine' movements, but only because it was asked of him by the professor who, by effecting the appearance of requiring only the quality of expression, tricked Jacques into carrying out graceful movement because he was 'obliged' to.

The injunction to perform and to perform well through artistic sublimation is of the same order as the religious sublimation at work when the goddess *Yemanja* or *Erzulie* possesses the body of the devotees, 'constraining' them to express a seductive and feline femininity which is not 'their own' and which they attribute to the divinity. In the same way that the faithful uses his body, not on his own account but in order to incarnate the Other under the form of the mythical entity, in dance therapy the subject expresses his desire under the 'veil' not of a god but of the gesture which he strives to render beautiful. The superego authorises such a sublimated transgression and Jacques was able to exorcise not only something of his repressed femininity, but also other repressed oedipal desires. He regulated, through ritualising and sublimation, the aggressiveness which was causing so many problems for his team of researchers. His hypochondriac complaints became more discrete, and he would even ask to join a group of dancers to work on a staged performance of Primitive Expression in which he experienced much success.

With sublimation, whether through analytical cure or dance therapy, our patient had arrived at the end of his therapeutic journey. Sublimation is thus the culmination of the course which we have attempted to retrace in this work, which leaves us with the question whether it constitutes the terminus of the adventure which has led the human being from animality to language and to embark on the quest for transcendence, or indeed whether it will lead to a new blossoming. The evolution of the human species is without doubt not yet terminated and could lead us along new and unexpected paths.

Amongst all the inventions of humanity, dance commemorates most joyfully and illustrates most fully the 'voyage' whose trajectory we have attempted to trace in this work, and which the dancer relives at all the levels which make up his existence. It is on such a foundation that rhythm dance therapy is built.

Notes

1 For example, the first drawings of the human child are tadpole-like figures, bereft of arms, which serves to accentuate their head, or perhaps their phallic meaning for the mother? Such is the impact of such an imaginary 'reality' that it is impossible to teach the child to represent it in terms which are not influenced by this glimpse into its own essence.
2 This report can be found in the article by France Schott-Billmann and Jean-Yves Collart in the journal *Art et Thérapie* No. 98/99 of February 2008 under the title 'Les dieux danseurs', pp. 27–36.
3 The Other: Language (i.e. = Culture, ancestors), but also Nature. The immortality of Nature, as well as language (Culture) explains why they are both capable of representing God. The other is the other human being.
4 Which we should understand in its most immediate sense: that the self is not complete in itself. It is 'lacking' something, namely the Other.

12 Rhythm dance therapy

According to the World Health Organization (WHO) we can define health as the state of equilibrium between the different levels which make up the human being: physical, social, mental and psychic. Dance constitutes a privileged therapeutic activity in so far as it integrates the body at the level of its motor functioning, the social at the level of the group link, and the psyche insofar as it awakens emotions and representations in an experience which is both symbolic and artistic.

Rhythm dance therapy (RDT) is developing rapidly in Europe and is today perceived by a growing number of practitioners as a particularly effective way of achieving the social and therapeutic objectives envisaged by dance therapy. It is taught at several associations in France: the *Société Française de Danse-thérapie* (SFDT, www.sfdt.free.fr) founded in 1984 which teaches it alongside other techniques, the *Atelier du geste rythmé* (www.gesterythme.com), founded in 1994, devoted to Primitive Expression and to *Danse Rythme Lien Social et Thérapie* (DRLST, www.drlst.org), while, since 2007, *ONG internationale* has offered Primitive Expression alongside other rhythmic activities such as popular, traditional and contemporary dance and music.

Rhythm dance therapy places rhythm at the core of its method. It bases itself theoretically on the human, social and clinical sciences, and its understanding of the nature and place of dance in RDT is, accordingly, the result of both an artistic and interdisciplinary enterprise. It rereads from a contemporary, multi-disciplinary perspective the social and therapeutic function of popular collective dances which for centuries took place in the village square during traditional festivals. It recalibrates these dances with contemporary expectations and employs them as a preliminary stage, serving to unite the group by awakening it to collective rhythm and preparing it thus to enter into the sphere of Primitive Expression.

Popular dances for therapeutic mediation

Next to traditional dance therapy (e.g. shamanism, possession) whose religious context restricts their application, a large range of dances are derived from our oral heritage: popular dances which are rhythmic and collective, offering expression through the body and helping to find a place within the greater whole (e.g. group, nature, the universe). They care by rendering vital, vibrant and resonating the relation of each individual to himself, his body, others and the environment.

While we may sometimes distinguish between popular art and the elite art of the upper classes, it would be more correct to see in them a difference in function: the former is concerned primarily with education (for all stages of life) and is present in all human society, whether or not they possess writing, a character which in no way contradicts its aesthetic dimension.

Yet dance therapy does not only consist in proposing dance technique, however beneficial and liberating. Dance with an explicitly therapeutic objective presupposes, without losing its artistic character, the ability to mediate between organiser (therapist) and public (patient).

The therapist

The therapist must be trained to help others and be capable of empathy. He must be prepared against the projections which cloud his perception of the dancers and the temptation to interpret their movements (which would give them no room for personal expression). He must know how to distance himself from his own subjectivity and efface himself as a person before the dance which constitutes a third person in the relationship. Only if all these conditions are met can dance play its role, offer its benefits and remain faithful to its therapeutic character, refined and matured over a long period by popular culture. In France, for example, dance therapy emerged during the 1950s with Rose Gaetner, a developmental therapist trained in dance, who worked with psychotic children in the day clinic *Santos-Dumont* in Paris. Her method, which was simple and intuitive, intimately linked music and dance according to traditional European dances. The participants formed a circle, in which the dance therapist proposed accessible movements to the accompaniment of music. The participants then repeated them together, each one according to their ability. No correction took place during the course of this transmission. Gaetner looked to the work of Wallon for the relationship between muscular tone and emotion as well as for the role of the mirror stage. She was also influenced by Ajurriaguerra's observations on the tonic psychomotor dialogue between mother and child, and Piaget concerning the structuring role of imitation in the constitution of the ego.

Rhythms belonging to oral culture

The forms of oral culture, whether traditional or modern (Zumthor, 1983: 182–202),[1] are marked by the regularity of the beat and the periodic return of the rhythm, in a movement which pulses between binary pairs. We speak of rhythmic music dance to designate those forms in which the beat, the rhythm and the movements are strongly and regularly marked.

Rhythm, which decisively structures the music forms of oral heritage, obeys an order which, emanating from the body itself, is entirely natural. Music and dance project its vital rhythms:

- the regular beat of the heart is transposed into music through pulsation and the striking of the dancers' feet on the ground; and
- breath is transposed into music through couples of phrases of equal duration and imprints its character on all forms of oral culture: verbal (poetry), musical and gestural. It endows them with the continuity of an irreducible inseparability of the body, music, voice and gesture.

It is, therefore, the body which imposes its order on the two 'twin sisters' of music and dance. It carries them and they carry it: they beat like the heart and respire like a sonorous and gestural projection of the ribcage. Popular dance is metaphoric by nature, yet profoundly incarnates life at its most profound level: heart, and breath. It is this organic system, musicalised, vocalised and gesturalised by the dancer, which is put to work in the therapeutic process. This often begins with a song chosen by the group from its own oral heritage. The flux of the voice in choral chant is not uniform, it is supported by a 'pulse', a punctuated, regular application of pressure which carves out paired melodic units modelled on the contraction and expansion of the respiratory system as it resonates through the voice. Organised as a projection of corporeal rhythms returned, as it were, to the outside, the musical forms of oral culture reflect back upon the exterior in reverse: as immaterial and sonorous. Music is an invisible, pulsating body.

Song

Listening to the 'voice' of music presents us from the outset with a certain number of surprises. Even seated, not to say lying down, participants almost always exhibit a corporeal reaction. It could be minimal or strong. It may take the form of a discrete movement (of the head or another part of the body, sometimes an extremity, a finger, toe, a light tap of the foot on the ground or hand on the thighs). Alternatively it may take the form of a rhythmic movement of the whole body which no longer seems capable of resting in place, as it has been carried away by the powerful and contagious surging of energy which the rhythm provokes. Each individual responds in his own way to the call addressed to him by the song. It awakens in him something which remains poised in expectation; and then starts to resonate, converting the music into a rhythmic movement of the body. The continuity between bodily and sonorous expression reminds us that dance and music were originally inseparable popular expressions (Zumthor, 1983: 196). The first sensation awakened by this experience so simple and yet so rich is that of an increase in energy coursing through the body: from the feet to the head or the head to the feet. We sense it everywhere, in the limbs and in the stomach, though we do not know its source. For many the effect it induces is akin to an itching sensation, a desire to move the legs. Those who can, stand up and dance; others discover that they can dance while sitting down.

The songs to which we dance constitute part of our oral heritage, transmitted without the intervention of writing, directly through the body. They embody a popular memory which binds men to one another, to their body, to their origins and to nature. They are the voice of the people abstracted from the vicissitudes of history: a corporeal voice, atemporal and universal, which in the pulsation of its rhythm speaks directly to the heart and carries a civilising message. Oral expression cannot be reduced to the voice; it involves the entire body in its relationality. Oral art is more than any other inseparable from the socially cohesive and stabilising function of art. Its harmony emanates from the very body of man and prepares him for entering into relation with others and with the world.

The mother transmits to the child the call of a voice which plunges into the night of time. The rhythmic structure of choral music (sung in choir) reactivates in each one the memory of their relation with the mother whose heart they heard beating while immersed in the amniotic fluid, accompanied by the periodic surge of her respiration. After birth, held against her chest, the child rediscovers this beating and when she rocks him to the rhythm of the cradle the breath of her voice literally enchants him (as Plato had already noticed in *The Laws* (VII: 790 d–e).[2] Is this harmonic, which couples two movements to make of them one, not the first dance, a dance for two, with the other first human, the mother? It is the primal experience of childhood which returns when the participants, whether standing or seated, sing and move together: the sensation of being stirred by a force exterior to the self which is the rhythmic voice of music. The regular beat brings body, rhythm and voice into synergy, giving access to the ancient, the deeply buried, the foetal experience whose prosody is marked by the beating of the heart of the mother and the expansion–retraction of respiration.

Belonging to the group

Clapping the hands and singing are fundamentally a group activity. The song precedes the dance and assembles the participants around a common rhythm. Its regular pulse beats out a series of points of orientation, structures of sharing. The participants find themselves in a profound synchrony: all are united in the joy of this sharing, in the enthusiasm for repetition which allows the flow of energy to increase. The stimulating, containing and reassuring sentiment of belonging to a group induces the famous 'letting go', while the barriers fall just as much inside the self as outside. Beings which are separated, solitary, cut off from their inner nature and from each other, discover themselves to be members of a common body. Sharing rhythm enables, according to the expression of Euripides, to 'put souls in common' by taking pleasure together in the feeling of being alive, by partaking in the soul of the festival.

An unconscious science

The measure of the voice chanted in a choir makes the self aware of the presence of latent forces and an unsuspected knowledge of rhythm, a knowledge installed in the body by the very mechanism which keeps us alive: the rhythm of the heart and respiration. No one pays attention to these internal movements, which maintain themselves without the intervention of the conscious will. Their transposition into music, however, is immediately recognised by the body and awakens a compulsion to move under the 'pressure' of its pulsation. Humming or whistling an unknown tune, clapping the hands and moving to the rhythm of the music: they all entail the joy of discovering in oneself a forgotten unconscious knowledge; yet one that is so readily available. The immediate transformation of the gaze and bearing of the individual testifies to this discovery of a hidden nature, one which is coded differently than the often disorientated social ego (Zumthor, 1983: 269). The dancer attains another reality which he feels is truer and more substantive than mundane reality insofar as through it, he is connected to the body, to others and to the group. He shares with those around him the joy of this recognition of self exceeding the individual and linking all within the flow of common energy.

The creative process

Winnicott's concept of found-created object is particularly useful when addressing the question of creativity, too often confused with improvisation. It is of little importance whether the form emanates from the self or is incorporated from the outside. In both cases, the therapeutic process involves creation which is, above all, the creation of meaning. In dance, this refers to the capacity to invest the self in the gesture, which repetition enables us to progressively inhabit. At first receptive, the dancer 'hears himself' through the voice of music and the gestures of dance, which both speak to him and of him. He thereby progressively acquires the capacity to 'say himself', becoming at the same time emitter and source in a dynamic of creation and re-creation.

It does not take a long career as a dance therapist to recognise that the same gesture proposed to a group is recreated by each individual, echoed in as many different ways as there are dancers present. The therapist learns to recognise the structuring moment in which the gesture becomes signifying, takes on meaning: then the dancer incarnates and irradiates Presence. Dance allows the dancer to let go, delivering himself from the severity of his superego. He is reconciled with his 'primitive' roots, his link to nature and the domain of the instincts. He plays without complex the tiger and bird, the hunter, the farmer, the warrior. Gestures and voices assume meaning and create meaning.

Joy

Do they move or are they moved when together the dancers acknowledge with their bodies the pulsating of the heart of music and the surging of its respiration? Singing the music, clapping hands and moving the body bring bodily and musical rhythms into phase. Who directs this choir: is it the rhythm of the heart which regulates that of the music or the reverse? The inside is externalised as if the music projected the sonorities of the ribcage onto the exterior, while the outside is interiorised when it permeates us, allowing us to sense our most buried corporeal rhythms. This reversibility of the couple inside/outside complements that of receptivity/activity: receptor/emitter, passive/active. The participant is in two states at the same time: he receives the music AND he acts it: he is moved AND he moves. This reversibility is the secret of trance: the movement takes place on its own. It is repeated without the requirement of thought to maintain it, as if the Other directed our body in our place. The Other celebrated in these dances is the living, hidden treasure of the oral heritage of humanity (Zumthor, 1983: 269).[3] They have conserved for millennia the secret of the traditional procedures for putting us into relation with the other (the neighbour) and the Other through trance.

The dance is not only directed towards human persons or concrete objects, the other with a small o, but rather aspires towards that which exceeds it: the Other. Whether we call it the divine, the sacred, the archetypes or the symbolic dimension (e.g. language, art, religion, science), the Other is alterity for man, his non-ego which attracts him irresistibly from the moment that he is born. Designated by Freud as sublimation, Lacan names it the 'invoking drive'.

The universal relation of dance to trance, throughout its variations unique to each culture in the richness of our popular heritage, indicates that access to trance was selected by evolution and maintained throughout the ages in recognition of its beneficial effects for groups and individuals. Yet the word trance continues to be the cause of fear in the West. The dance therapist accordingly prefers to speak of enthusiasm, or to employ a word which fortunately is returning to conferences on dance therapy: joy.[4] We have adopted this word, shared by all who have embraced the profession of dance therapist; yet let us not forget that the state of forgetfulness of self is the principal therapeutic factor. It is always this forgetfulness, the principal means of access to the Other, which is sought after, whether or not this goal is explicitly acknowledged. Dancers incarnate the mystery of life, the biological and psychic together, which they celebrate in group form, communing with its sources as with other dancers, participating with them in the Living. Without conscious action, all kinds of energetic or symbolic processes, which are mysteriously reparative, come into play at is behest; since they are the guardians of life.

Rhythm dance therapy using Primitive Expression

Popular traditional dances are not to everyone's taste, neither are more contemporary forms of oral expression (e.g. rock, disco, techno, rap). Yet how can RDT reject such a groundswell which has since the start of the twentieth century given to popular dance its overwhelmingly cosmopolitan and intercultural character? I have chosen a dance of more recent creation, which is both traditional and contemporary insofar as it undergoes perpetual recreation: Primitive Expression. It possesses the advantages of popular dances (accessibility, energy, joy, communication, link to the group, liberation of the body, harmony of movement and spatiotemporal structuring) reinforced by its 'primitive' character which renders it more simple, powerful and attractive to our contemporary society sensitive to the aesthetic of the 'first' arts. The result is a very physical dance to a powerful rhythm with expansive gestures: a dance without borders, drawing from various sources in a trans-cultural spirit which bears witness to both the unity and diversity of humanity.

It can boast in particular of a rich and varied imagination, seeking to give expression to our relation to nature, animal heritage, ancestral activities and traditional crafts. It enables us to experience them within an atmosphere which is both warm and playful, excluding neither emotion nor the relation to the Other.

Primitive Expression inherited the insights gained from Katherine Dunham's research and participation in the trance rituals of the Caribbean (especially Haitian *vaudoo*) during which divinities descend 'into the body' of the devotees and make them dance. We have replaced the gods with archetypes (symbols which speak to everyone: children and adults, the sick and healthy, without distinction of nationality or social group) and religious transcendence, sacred experience with artistic sublimation. Each one can find in them not only meaning, but also a veritable experience of self.

Therapeutic tools in Primitive Expression

The rhythm dance therapist, as the name suggests, must possess multi-disciplinary training. He must put his artistic knowledge at the service of his function, have acquired knowledge in the domain of the social and clinical sciences and possess the qualities of a good organiser. He must equally be trained in therapy and have himself experienced the therapeutic process as participant.

The strong therapeutic potential of Primitive Expression derives from its rhythmic structures and symbolic armoury. We must nevertheless deconstruct and re-adapt it according to contemporary needs and tastes. Rhythm dance therapists should also be trained to take inspiration from the rhythmic games played between mother and child and ritual as a reservoir of poetic sign images capable of awakening the imagination while containing the drives. We must finally instil in practitioners the ethics underlying this mode of care.

Let's look at these three points.

Between tradition and modernity: a playful deconstruction

On the basis of popular and tribal dances, Primitive Expression perceives the rhythmic structures which from the start activate and bring into relation beat, repetition and symmetry. It accentuates the element of play which is the royal road to therapy (Winnicott, 2005).

The process of deconstruction which Primitive Expression employs seeks to strip away all traces of folklore to attain to a more minimalist, sober and powerful form of dance. A parallel deconstruction of accompanying music leads to the use of rhythmic fundamentals (played often on the *djembé*). We are here continuing the work of Katherine Dunham and her deconstruction of the complexities of Caribbean dances, classical dance and popular European dances with a view to reconstructing elementary rhythmic structures of beat and binarity. Movements are organised according to a division of time (i.e. 8, 4, 2 or 1) which is nothing other than the application in music and dance of the principle of 'split representation' characteristic, according to Lévi-Strauss, of the primitive arts. This minimalism in rhythmic organisation brings the dancer as close as possible to the bodily rhythms of the cardiac pulsation and the expansion–contraction of breath. It branches into the vital mechanisms: the heart and breath transpose themselves into its movement and repeat their own within it as if automatically. Dancing between nature and culture, the beat of the music awakens the pulse, activating an energy which is half-corporeal, half-psychic.

Deconstruction applies also to gestures. Arms which are not occupied with contact with another partner as in popular dances can be used to sculpt simple forms in space: sharp, powerful, stylised; forms which are purified and, in similar terms to primitive art as Picasso understood it, in turn, capable of purifying us. The repetition of gestures is a powerful inducer of trance. It transforms the initial movement, which is confused, inhibited and charged with anxiety, liberating it progressively from its blockages and parasites, and re-orientating it positively (like the drives through the analytical cure). It enables the gesture to affirm itself in its pure essence, free from the excess of emotional charge which encumbers it, giving it access thereby to the domain of the universal.

The deconstruction of the voice which accompanies the gestures lightens it of its semantic burden. It becomes a pure vocal rhythmic or melodic game which uses bare phonemes, in themselves disconnected from words.

The principles of rhythmic games

The rhythm dance therapy of Primitive Expression locates itself at the intersection between the human, clinical and social sciences within the framework of a multidimensional project which seeks to ground 'scientifically' the therapeutic function of dance through rhythmical games organised following anthropological and psychological laws.

Symbolic function

The anthropologist (Lévi-Strauss) and psychoanalysis (Freud) both insist on the necessary role which symbolisation plays in the process of acceding to our humanity. The human being, after all, is the only animal capable of symbolising (i.e. linking) a signifier to a signified. Becoming human involves a wide-ranging renunciation of the satisfaction of the instincts, including the delusion of being all powerful, by obliging them to flow into symbolic moulds which both socialise them and render them communicable.

The symbolic function implies, therefore, both the renouncing of the simple discharge of the drive and the capacity to establish a meaning underlying an object or gesture, which is capable of evoking both the concrete (a thing) and abstract (an idea or emotion). This function is also necessary to the maintenance and re-establishing of psychic equilibrium. Whether preventative or curative, the therapeutic process consists, according to the Freudian model, in finding representations for those affects which are pathogenic because they have not been, or only badly, symbolised.

The mechanism of symbolisation involves the subject in a bipolar rhythm linking signifier and signified. The rhythmic structures, whose oscillation the body of the dancer traces through the dimensions of space, reach towards the foundations of the person. It is not surprising, therefore, that they are prevalent in the practices of traditional oral societies, nor that they can be rediscovered in all the forms enabling us to revisit and consolidate the psychological foundations of human existence.

The humanising law: differentiation

Claude Lévi-Strauss underlines the universality of the two great civilisatory interdictions: incest and murder. They are transmitted from generation to generation as a 'natural law' governing the family. They imply both the renouncing (i.e. the confusion–fusion of incest, and all the confusions) and an authorisation (i.e. the search for a distanced partner according to separation–differentiation). This natural law, transmitted tacitly to the child by the parents, rests on the distinction of categories differentiated according to binary opposition: masculine/feminine, individual/collective, child/parent, authorised/forbidden, pure/impure, family/society, etc. Differentiation, which is opposed to fusion, is at the foundation of the construction of society as well as of the individual. Psychology stresses that an acknowledgement of the interdiction against incest or murder is an indispensable structuring element in the development of the child in its passage from the Oedipus stage, a stage during which it feels love towards one parent and dreams of eliminating the other. We know the psychic damage which results from the all-too-frequent transgression of this interdiction inducing in the victim a generalised confusion, not only between the generations which should remain sexually distant, but between all categories of opposites: fantasy and reality, the imagination and symbolic, and so on.

One of the functions of oral tradition, whose aim is to educate and socialise, is precisely to transmit this civilising law. It does this in discrete and playful fashion through the rhythmic practices at the heart of different artistic expressions: music, poetry, narrative, theatre, all rooted in the activity of children and marked by the seal of a rhythm perceived during the first vocal, mimic and gestural exchanges which babies have with those around them (Schott-Billmann, 2001: 114–116).

Parental functions

Parents traditionally educate the child via the operation of two functions. The maternal function is nourishing, containing, reassuring, and takes place within a relation of corporeal proximity to the child. It is necessary to endow the latter with the force required to separate. The paternal function serves progressively to create distance from the mother in order to lead the child towards society (and in the same movement to separate opposites).

156 *The therapeutic process*

The work of Jacques Lacan, who recognised willingly his debt to Lévi-Strauss, enables us to establish an important link between anthropology and psychoanalysis. Aware of the necessary role of the humanising Law in the exiting of the state of fusion, Lacan refers it to the paternal function, which we have also observed at work in the 'Nom du Père'.

Given the close parallel between the work of the mother and of the therapist (Stern, 1985), the latter must also play a maternal and paternal role. Like the mother, he seeks to reassure the patient in his basic narcissism, while like the father, leading towards differentiation, autonomy, expression, and the harmonious, balanced link between all the opposites constitutive of the human being (e.g. body and mind, drives and representations, masculine and feminine, etc.) (Stern, 1985). As such, he presides over the relation between self and other (neither too close nor too distant).

An anthropological ritual

Celebrating our origin returns the 'primitive' imagination to the surface, a Real which has become largely silent in our era. The ritual of Primitive Expression is capable of bringing to expression and harnessing this Real through a festival of song and dance, one which is both playful and poetic; a celebration which is anthropological, insofar as it revisits the sources of humanisation, and ecological insofar as it mediates our relation to nature.

The call of the drum awakens the flowing, Dionysian energy which has its source in the rhythms of the body and the vital energy. It is a fundamental aspect of primitive expression, and is a precious aid in the treatment of depressives or asthenics. The original vital rhythms transposed into the sound of the drum, transfuse the dancer with an energy which surprises him. It courses through all his being: his head, his stomach and feet. It pulses through his body like blood through his veins. Under the effect of this pressure, of its compulsion which is at the same time an invocation, the dancer feels the urgent need to express a flowing, violent, instinctual energy. It finds its outlet in the stamping of the feet, but it also searches forms into which it can flow and which are capable of regulating it. The participants express the rhythm through an impetuous leaping forwards, backwards, to the right, to the left and a turning around on the spot; then in joyous rhythmic greetings shared between all members of the group, before celebrating their common relation to the universe through gestures symbolizing their relation to the earth and the mysterious link which ties them to the cosmos. They greet the four cardinal points, invoking the sky and the earth (Figure 12.1).

Now symbolically linked to the world around them, the participants are invited to perform 'archetypal' symbolic gestures. Primitive Expression makes it possible to access the archaic memory; to enter a kind of dream-state where all sorts of unconscious healing processes, energising or symbolic, come into play-giving life (Roustang, 2008). They discover a knowing-dancing close to natural movement, an ancient wisdom of the body which they did not know they possessed. Caught up in life's movement, abandoned to the rhythm, delivered from the severity of

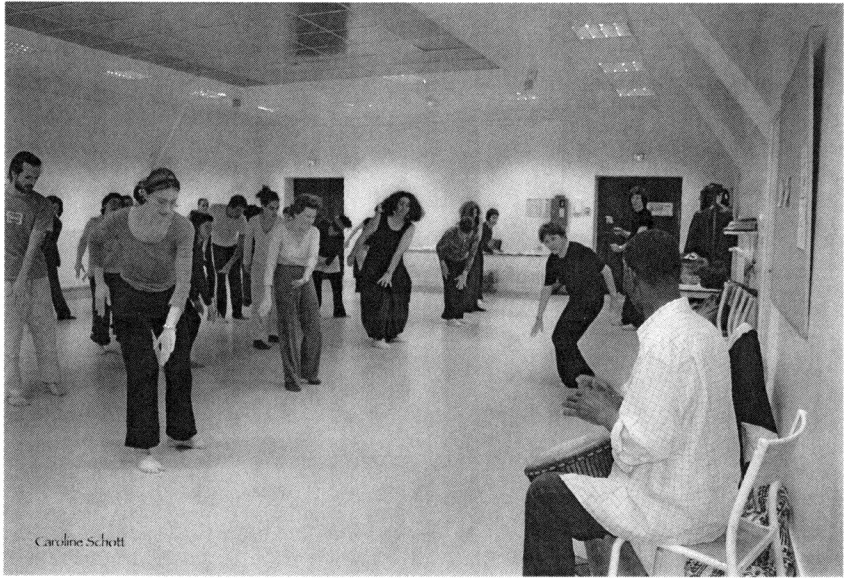

Figure 12.1 The call of the drum: Henri Samba and hailing the Earth
Source: Photo by Caroline Schott

the superego by letting go, the dancers play the tiger or bird, the hunter, the cultivator, or the warrior . . . without any complex. The gesture is freed little-by-little from its blockages and negative elements, is positively reoriented, as the unconscious drive in an analytical cure, to be affirmed in its pure essence, purified of egotistical emotions that weigh it down, and thus attain a universal dimension (Figure 12.2).

Mimesis, in such a context, involves neither a passive attitude nor a submissive act, but a profound experience of renewal, of self-representation, of self re-creation and of transformation. The experienced therapist knows how to recognise this structuring moment because the gesture is lived, is incarnated: it takes on both meaning and presence.

This unsuspected knowledge, flowing from a source deep within the dancer, serves to channel and order raw movement through rhythm. At the same time, it brings the different parts of the body into harmony and the different levels of human existence (e.g. physical, social, mental psychic) into shared resonance and into equilibrium. The World Health Organization defines this as the standard for establishing and maintaining a good state of health.

Primitive Expression seeks to tie together the natural and symbolic by framing the successive mobilising of the different parts of the body in terms of a symbolism which opens the dancer to a creative process. The body and the gesture become bearers of meaning. The dancer is offered gesture-images: representations of

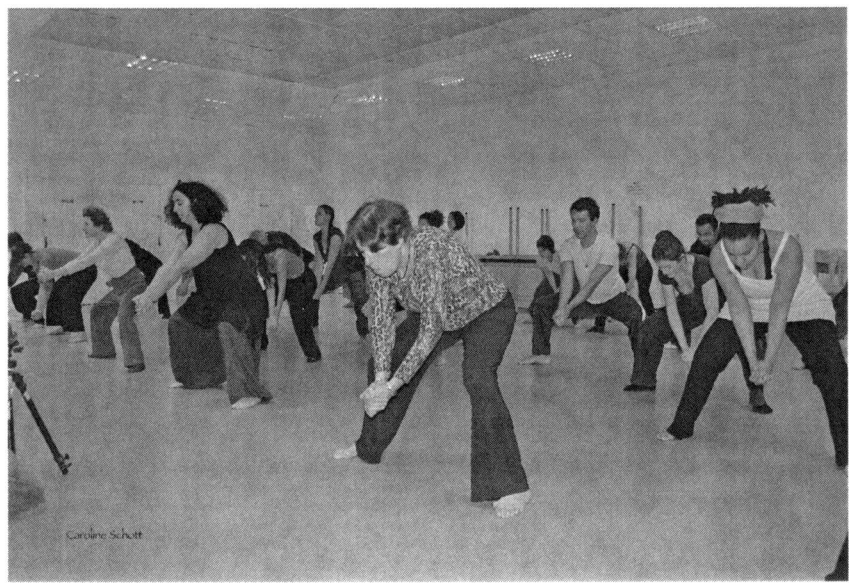

Figure 12.2 Finding the ancestral gesture
Source: Photo by Caroline Schott

actions, animals and characters to act, a musical score to interpret. He captures them mimetically, repeating and appropriating them towards the end of his own self-expression, and executes them to increasing levels of speeds punctuated with stops which 'crystallise' the movement into a posture, transform it into a statue. It is during these 'stops' that the body assumes a precise form, one which can be represented, communicated and observed by the other.

Ethics

His knowledge of psychology allows the rhythm-dance therapist to adapt his work to his audience. His choice of dance, whether from our oral heritage or Primitive Expression, etc., will be determined by the public he has before him. He will not ask the aged or adolescents to strictly follow all the formalities of dance. Neither will he push the anorexic towards mastery of their body; he will rather lead him towards abandon, a letting-go, towards pleasure, because he is aware of his hypercontrol and the persistence of the feeling of being powerful which he harbours. He will not encourage the hysteric to excess but will offer them the possibility, through gesture, to channel their emotions. He will help the obsessive to liberate themselves from obedience to the superego by avoiding any imposition of a rigid framework.

His personal therapeutic approach will prepare him to deal with the effects of the transfer of the participants and to be alert to the risk of his own countertransference. In this quest for the self, the psychoanalytical approach is privileged. This is because, on the one hand, of its homology to the process of deconstruction which, as we have seen, is central to our method and on the other hand, because it allows the therapist to deconstruct in equal measure his illusory personalities as they manifest themselves on the couch and those which attach parasitically to his movements in dance. As such, it allows the therapist to efface himself behind the gesture which he proposes. This attitude of discretion resembles that of the psychoanalyst who maintains a low profile so as not to encumber this person with that which initiates the process of the cure.

The rhythm dance therapist trusts in the dance and in its rhythmic structures which have survived for millennia. He integrates them into his propositions and incites them to play the role of the third, the mediator in the relationship. He will let music call the dancer, and he will leave it to the dancer to acknowledge and repeat the gesture in his own way. We may refer to Lacan here who, on the basis of linguistic concepts, distinguishes the received form from its expression in a style which is unique to each one: it is in the expression that the unconscious desire of the subject manifests itself.

Through his double training in dance and psychotherapy, the rhythm dance therapist has learned the necessity of respecting the mystery of the unconscious. He knows that there is the Real, an indecipherable which must be tolerated, and which music and dance enable us to hear and feel. Dance therapy is a profound experience of the renewal, transformation and re-creation of self. It allows us to take the Real from its unexpressed, unperceived, unheard state and give it form in the musical movement of dance. At first invoked, the self becomes the invoker (calling the Other in its turn); at first recipient of the collective enouncement, it will become the emitter of his own vocal and gestural enunciation, one which inscribes his singularity in the universal.

Refraining from making 'interpretations' of art

Is the therapist required to interpret the productions of the patient and take account of them in his treatment? For my own part, I do not practise the 'reading' of the body in dance therapy; I prefer to listen to the gestural discourse of the patient within the framework of transfer: which is say, addressed to the therapist. A movement of weak amplitude and little energy should not be seen in terms of an 'emotional blockage' resulting from the history of the subject or his character defences; rather in terms of a message sent to the therapist, such as 'I fear you who remind me of my mother' or 'I am afraid of having the desire to kill, so I am holding myself back', etc. The therapist must then attempt to 'hear' and 'respond' through the attitude he takes towards the patient or by proposing a new action. If he is a good listener and possesses good clinical sense, the assistance offered by the art therapist may constitute not simply an adjunctive treatment but also a therapeutic intervention in its own right. Certainly it is not a question here of acting like the classical therapist. It is precisely one of the pitfalls of the latter, one of its deviations, not to say perversions, to forget the unique character of such treatment and 'psychologise' it. We refuse to take this step in dance whose wealth and therapeutic power vastly exceed the framework of the explicit expression of contents. Dance is at one and the same time link, framework, unification of the body, and 'structurisation' of the psyche. A psychologising interpretation (e.g. 'the character of your walk is symptomatic of your problems with your mother') of the kind which takes place too often through a 'reading of the body', is at best partial, reductive and defensive, if not totally inadequate.

Something in art escapes psychological analysis: it aspires to go beyond all limits. As we observed in our consideration of repetition, the movement of 'going further' is constitutive of human desire itself. It appears, therefore, from the start driven by the search for what Freud called 'sublimation', which is a crucial aspect of art therapy and represents the last link in the chain of the process leading the human from animality to speech. It indeed goes further, driving towards the emergence through art of a Presence which appears to exceed the human register and which we will refer to as the sublime (which etymologically signifies beyond all limits).

In shamanism (as in psychoanalysis) and dance we do not know what heals us: it is when we are occupied with something else, transported, the spirit elsewhere, in a state of trance, that without our knowledge, through the dynamism of the symbol (spoken or danced), the reorganisation which transforms our life takes place. It must remain secret because superfluous words and commentaries will only see it slip from our grasp. Symbolic efficacy is delicate and requires the veil of poetry, rhythm, dance and music. Under the veil, art works to heal us, while preventing us, according to the beautiful expression of Nietzsche, from 'dying from the truth'.

Notes

1 Traditional orality (e.g. poetry, songs, popular dance, nursery rhythms, lullabies, etc.) are making a comeback today in new contemporary forms, (e.g. rap, slam, rock, etc.) which exhibit the same rhythmic structures within a musical patchwork which brings into continuity music, poetry and dance.
2 'When mothers want to lull their restless children to sleep, they do not provide stillness but just the opposite, motion; they rock them constantly in their arms, and not with silence but with some melody. It is exactly as if they were charming the children. . . .'
3 What UNESCO today calls immaterial heritage: the ensemble of traditions and endangered cultures, technical crafts and living artistic expressions. Paul Zumthor speaks of 'oraliture', which he opposes to 'literature'.
4 Margariti Alexia, et al., 'An application of the Primitive Expression form of dance therapy in a psychiatric population', *The Arts in Psychotherapy* 39 (2), 95–101, 2012.

13 New fields in the application of rhythm dance therapy

We would like to close this study into the therapeutic efficacy of dance by giving an outline of its application within new fields. Dance therapy has left its ivory tower far behind: the diversity of its workshops and adaptability of its practices testify to its vitality and relevance in the treatment of some of the most acute problems we face today, not only in the clinical, but also in the social, political and cultural domain.

We have chosen two workshops: the first can broadly located within the social field (dances for peace in Israel), the other in the field of handicap (Parkinson's disease). We will strive to capture not only the method but also the atmosphere essential to dance therapy. It is not, after all, a question simply of technique, but also of fostering interrelation. These two workshops will allow us to see the method of DRLST (dance, rhythm, social link and therapy) at work, which searches above all to awaken vital rhythmic sources by inviting participants to share in practices drawn from oral tradition (e.g. popular songs, lullabies, rhymes, raps . . .) and to lead them towards a reliving of the experience of the earliest rhymes and the rhythmic relation to the other.

The social field and dancing for peace

Restoring the social link is an essential objective of the most recent form of dance therapy, Primitive Expression. It is founded on the belief that rhythmic oral practices, whether traditional or revisited by modernity, are capable of offering us new ways of responding to the contemporary impasse insofar as they turn us towards new forms of relation, mending the tears in our social fabric. Through DRLST, moreover, dance therapy has turned itself anew towards the social realm, to the streets of our cities. It has embarked on a voyage which has profoundly modified the face of classical art therapy and cultivated an international network of enthusiastic practitioners immersed in culture, art and therapy, while being profoundly socially engaged.

When we start to entertain the role of dance beyond national boundaries, we find that we must respond to a new question: if rhythm offers a means for bringing down the interior walls of the individual self, or indeed between selves, could it not also have the same effect between people? This thought has given birth to a new dream: the application of dance therapy within the sphere of politics under the rubric of 'Dancing for Peace'.

Dancing for peace in Israel

Dances, which in their strongly regular and rhythmic character recall the beating of the heart and the surging of the pulse, are at the service of life and therefore of peace. They cultivate vivacity, confidence and openness to others; their rhythmic structures carry within them the power to bind together. If dance can makes barriers fall not only within the interior of the self, but also between individuals, even between groups, rhythm dance therapy (RDT) might offer a human, artistic bridge between self and other, a link between communities which counteracts their reciprocal isolation and self-enclosure.

The project

Whilst reflecting on how to apply the linking power of rhythm to the wider scale of entire peoples, the idea was forged of proposing dance workshops for peace to members of communities in conflict. It was hoped that these would help to sow 'the seeds of reconciliation' between people.

The frustrating pace of political negotiations and the failure of dialogue have led many to expect little from governments and to imagine solutions rising from below rather than dictated from above. To this end, I met Ayelet Ranen, a rhythm dance therapist in Israel and conceived with her the programme 'Dance of peace, dance of the heart'.[1]

The title serves to recall that there is in dance a trans-cultural structure which is not bound by the caprices of history: its pulsing rhythm, the heart of music and dance, can be recognised the world over. Common to all, it is neither Israeli nor Palestinian, neither Jewish nor Muslim nor Christian: it belongs to humanity. The same pulse animates the music and dance of numerous cultures where popular oral tradition has been preserved. We also find it in the songs and dances of Israelis and Palestinians, so we imagined that this common denominator could play a mediating role between two cultural groups as it did in America in linking the musical heritages of African and American culture from jazz to rock and its derivatives today, rap and techno.

I wanted to go to Israel to offer Palestinians and Jews, without expecting any miracle, the possibility of sharing a concrete experience: that of leaving behind binary thinking, of detaching for a while from the feeling of belonging to one or the other culture.

Within the context of conflict between two communities, we considered the technique of Primitive Expression to be the most judicious choice. It allows people to forget cultural difference, bringing participants together around its 'beat', acoustically close to the beating of the heart. It renders the dance reassuring and integrating, offering security, transition and exchange and therefore rendering possible a glimpsing, beyond the resentment which poisons the everyday life of the two communities, of a co-existence which is perhaps more 'natural' to being human.

We strongly insisted on not emphasising difference, concentrating rather on commonality and sharing via a form of dance which is not bound by any frontiers and which might therefore serve as a mediating third. There are many involved in Israel in the search for peace who agree that a non-verbal inter-cultural activity possesses the advantage of being able to accomplish a 'natural' rapprochement of peoples, whereas the use of language is marked from the outset by difference, all the more so in the state of Israel where Hebrew is the official language as much for Jews as for Arabs.

We wanted, however, to go further, proposing a trans-cultural form of dance which would offer a symbol for a possible future in which peace would represent not only the absence of war, but also the sharing of something which transcends differences and which constitutes the ancestral heritage of humanity, that which makes us human.

The programming of the atelier was made easier by the fact that France is perceived in this region, rightly or wrongly, as a neutral country. This fact assures its citizens a more favourable reception when acting in the role of mediator. Nevertheless, the realisation of the project would not have been possible without the combined efforts of a number of people engaged in the search for peace: Ayelet Ranen, indefatigable dance therapist, an Israeli trained in Paris at the Atelier du geste rythmé, Dr Eldad Pardo, an Islamologist, and Shelley Elkayam, a poet, both of whom are researchers attached to the Truman Institute for Peace at the Hebrew University of Jerusalem. They were able to interest the director of Theatrical Studies, Professor Moraly in our project, who, in turn, gave us access to a practice room.

It was agreed that Ayelet Ranen would assist me, translate (into Hebrew) and film the session. A percussionist, Daniel Feingold, would accompany the workshop, and a photographer Uri Noymeir, appointed by Professor Moraly, would take images, as was the practice in the Hebrew University each time a workshop for peace took place, which generally speaking, did not often involve dance!

The workshop

The first workshop took place on 3 February 2008 in Jerusalem. The university had been closed for the previous two days due to snow, so few students received the information displayed in Hebrew and Arabic on different panels and doors. Despite this, we received over 20 participants.

Amongst the students I counted five Palestinians from the West Bank, a young Arab Muslim from East Jerusalem, 11 Israeli Jews and some foreigners (from the USA, Australia and France). There were also university representatives (the two researchers who had first invited me) and three care professionals (a teacher, therapist and social worker). They formed a mixed group, as much in terms of culture as religion (four young girls from Ramallah, Muslim Palestinians, who wore the veil, another young girl from Palestine who did not wear the veil, as well as Jews and Christians) as in terms of studies pursued (political sciences, law, psychology, educational science, theatre, ITC). A diverse number of universities were also represented. Among others, we were joined by a Palestinian student with a diploma in psychology from the University of Beir Zeit, students of theatre trained in the French method of Jacques Lecoq and in American techniques, as well as students hailing from literature and the sciences.

I tried my best not to be overly worried at the thought that these participants, seated in a circle and about to present themselves to each other, were expecting something tangible, a concrete result, from this initiative. The young Palestinian women sat side by side together, timid and silent, coming to experience for the first time a dance of this kind. Then there were others who were already more or less disabused of any utopian notions regarding what could be expected from this kind of workshop.

Given such diversity, what commonality could I rely on to initiate the process which was to culminate in the mediating agent of Primitive Expression? My fears made me doubt what I was doing there. Why not simply allow them to dance their own dances? Yet how was I to avoid falling into cultural nationalism?

The first dance: the lullaby

I proposed starting at the beginning. I began with that which makes us all human, what the mothers all over the world over transmit to their children directly through their body, through the rhythmic movement of oral expression: the lullaby. To prepare for the listening I recalled that this is also the first dance which we learn, while in the arms of the mother. This stirred a certain emotion in the audience, accentuated through listening to an Arab lullaby ('Naami Naami') then to a Jewish lullaby sung in Yiddish ('Lialkele lialkele ay lu-lu') recorded on a CD of world music. The experiences attached to such songs, so old that we believed them forgotten, are in reality unforgettable, since the feelings which they stirred return so strongly to the surface.

Moving in common, sharing an emotion, recognising oneself through the mirror of the others, creating a reciprocal echoing together with the others, existing in a state of common sympathy (which etymologically signifies suffering together): is it not the foundation of the link to the other? Moreover, hearing a lullaby chanted by a feminine voice awakens a particular emotion: a wave of tenderness tinged with nostalgia, stronger, without doubt, in the Mediterranean context where the evocation of the mother, who has a privileged affective status, does not go without a certain sadness of the separation which, in this region, immediately evokes the separation imposed by history from the birth of the state of Israel.

Ouafa, a Palestinian woman who lives in Neve-Shalom,[2] spoke of her sadness on hearing this song, which she had heard before in Lebanon, a country which is now forbidden to all Israeli citizens, whatever their ethnic or religious origin. Everyone in the group suffered from the isolation from neighbouring regions imposed on their people. The lullaby heard together led them experience a new sensation, one which was known by all yet which had to be uncovered because it was felt at the most profound level of the body: the experience of love and separation recalled by the lullaby is both singular and shared. Anita, a Jewish woman of Neve Shalom, confided to us that this experience allowed her for the first time to associate the Arab language with a feeling other than fear. The hearing of the lullaby, she said, had allowed her to grasp something which evoked in her a Semitic, common world.

The lullaby reactivates the transitional space and the cluster of memories of the experience through which the child attains subjectivity. We consider it forgotten; yet it is just buried; when it comes back to the surface it awakens in us a state of openness and hopefulness. The fact of having accepting like a child the comforting rocking of the mother (that of one's own and of another) brings participants to the memory of a time before conflict: the time of the first exchange with another human, where nothing has yet taken place, allowing us to believe that things could have been otherwise; indeed still could be.

A common quality: sense of rhythm

Our relation to each other crossed a certain threshold when, standing together in a circle and holding each other by the hand, we allowed ourselves to rock together to the two lullabies. Beyond their differences in language and musical style, the first lullaby was nostalgic, the second dynamic. Through both, the swaying motion common to all lullabies entered our bodies, making of us one body moving to the music and being moved by the music. It rocked each one of us, as the mother rocked the child. Both rocked and rocking, we were all carried along by the waves of tenderness which the two singers conveyed to us, the living flux of song carried by the rhythmic surging of their voices. In this moment of regression, Plato came to mind: when the mothers sing a lullaby 'it is exactly as if they were charming the children . . .' (Plato, *The Laws,* VII, 790d–790e). We also were charmed, enchanted: bathing in the consolation of the group illusion; rediscovering something of the maternal body in which the child is suspended like a raft adrift on the amniotic ocean, in continuity with the liquid in state of 'oceanic feeling'.

The sharing of time: synchrony

Each one rocked to the music in their own unique fashion like a tree in the wind: present and alert; yet each one in his imaginary world, many of us with our eyes closed.

It was time to bring Primitive Expression into play to establish an inter-individual relation. The percussionist began to play the djembé, beating out a rhythm. The participants assembled around him and clapped their hands to this rhythm. This simple but collective response permitted the establishing of synchrony, a sharing of time which became a common reference. This sharing of time founded a solid inter-human link through rhythmic accord (Stern, 1985).³

Accompanied softly by the percussion, we began to sing together the lullaby 'Naami Naami' which possessed the advantage of existing in both languages. While clapping our hands, we also marked the rhythm with our feet and continued to sing (why deprive the body of its voice any more than of its movement?). Then we returned to form a circle, accelerating the rhythm while remaining in synchrony, united by the tempo. The participants would later report their joy at succeeding so easily in this activity and in sharing their success. I myself remarked on one quality common to all involved and which transcended their cultural differences: their excellent sense of rhythm, an aptitude which came naturally to them; yet which is less widespread among the inhabitants of more northerly countries. This observation seems to touch them deeply. After they had spread around the room, I invited them to walk to the rhythm, and then stand still upon the interruption of the music. With all subject to the same law, the law of time, they began to play, to exchange complicit glances, to smile when encountering one another.

The experience of a common support

The universal element shared by all men is the body. We can use it in dance therapy to cultivate a feeling of physical similarity (which is particularly marked among these two Semite peoples). This, in turn, can be used to cultivate a feeling of fraternity. Dance offers forms which translate into spatial terms: the characteristics of the body common to all human beings. We experienced this in Jerusalem. Standing in a circle and stamping their feet on the ground, the participants sang 'Naami Naami' together while moving back and forth to the rhythm of respiration and according to the three fundamental planes: 8 steps in front, 8 behind (sagittal plane), 8 steps to the right, 8 to the left (frontal plane), 8 steps to make a right turn, 8 for a left turn (horizontal plane). That day, in Jerusalem we were surprised, indeed astonished, to discover the ease with which such fundamentals were applied and shared. It is evident that these invariant structures have their root not only in the body, but also in the most profound levels of the psyche and remain present in the corporeal memory of each one, as a knowledge which is hidden in the real. Music and dance open the possibility of bringing them to expression.

I asked the percussionist to accelerate the tempo. The dancers followed without difficulty, carried by the rhythm of the group. They moved together, their joy and mounting energy clearly visible. The photographer strove to capture the intensity of this movement which was, as he would later remark, palpable in the atmosphere of the room. Might not the reason for this lie in the exhilaration induced by the 'sonorous (and I would add bodily) manifestation of an original phenomena of instinctual 'surging' and of the relation which unites instinct and joy (Lollo, 2007: 61)?

A common origin

I proposed Primitive Expression as a third party, mediating, dance. I first gave an historical presentation, explaining that it had originated likewise within a situation of conflict, although, of course, on another continent, America, where two communities existed in a state of tension with one another: African Americans and 'white' Americans. The dance was inspired by American choreographer, Katherine Dunham, herself the child of an African-American father and a French Canadian mother. She rediscovered the sources of Afro-American dance by observing Afro-Caribbean culture achieving a superimposition of common rhythmic structures, those precisely of the first, 'primitive' rhythms: beating and swaying. I explained that participants relive collectively what is common to all humanity: the musical and choreographic transposition of the rhythms of the heart and of breath; the use of the voice (chanted rhythmically yet without words, a series of phonemes belonging to no language); the harnessing of characteristics of the human body with its verticality, its cruciform structure and its symmetry which also organise its psychic construction (in terms of reflexivity, division of the subject, and relation to the other).

Revisiting the first rhythms and the foundations of the corporeal schema reactivates the original experience in which the child strives towards humanisation, and reawakens the memory of the first exchanges with another human being, the mother, leading the child from the natural rhythms felt within the womb (e.g. the beating of the heart and the drawing of breath) to the cultural rhythms (e.g. lullabies, songs, rhythmic games of alternation, imitation, call–response) which further structure their relationship. Shared rhythm is the humanising experience *par excellence*. It culminated on this occasion in a veritable instinctual revitalisation, a moment of intense happiness and healing. Against the backdrop of the war and death which plague the region in which we found ourselves on that day, this affirmation of life took on the fullest possible meaning, the supremacy of Eros over Thanatos.

Symbolic gestures

On that day in Jerusalem, what meaning could we perceive in the gestures through which we ritually greeted each other, cleared the branches which blocked our path, broke the trunks of trees, flew like a bird and hunted like a tiger, repulsed the demons and attracted the angels (common figures to the two cultures), passed through a tunnel opening out onto the light, replayed the invention of fire by our common ancestor by creating sparks, breathing on them and making them burst into flames? In any case, the level of energy, concentration and gravity invested by the participants in all of these gestures was remarkable. Their intensity and, dare we say it, love reached a height when in 4, 2 then 1 time, everyone together sent a message of peace in all directions of space (Figure 13.1).

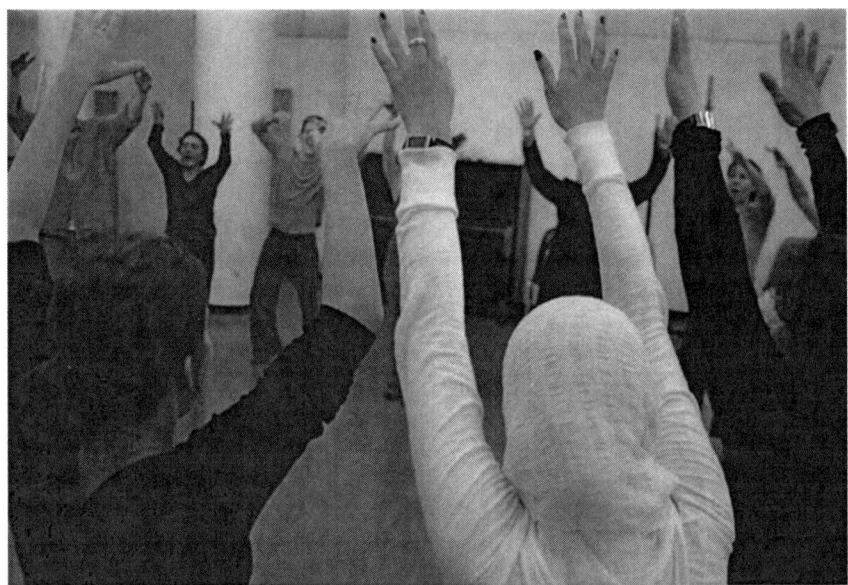

Figure 13.1 Sharing the rhythm in Jerusalem
Source: Photo by Uri Noymeier

The ritual concluded with an adaptation of a famous pre-monotheistic dance from Turkey, in which the dancers branch themselves into the movement of the rotation of the planets: the dance of the whirling dervishes.

Group and individual creativity

Afterwards, a collective improvisation of free dance allowed us to dance together to the rhythm of percussion; yet each one according to their style, eastern or western. We were now in a position to display and offer to one another our cultural differences after assuring ourselves of our common foundation. We could thus, without danger, live both similarly to and differently from each other, and discover how much differences can be enriching and complementary at the cultural level where they can be expressed within an atmosphere of attentiveness and respect.

Sharing the same rhythm, the entire group in synchrony, fraternal in being subject to the same rhythmic law, a law which is applied equally to all yet endowing each in its movement with their freedom, their own singularity and style: does this not constitute an exemplary pre-figuration of a society in which the rights of man reign over all, an equality, fraternity and liberty so joyously accepted and respected in dance?

The workshop, which lasted four and half hours, came to an end with the creation of dances of peace carried out in small groups of four or five people composed of mixed nationalities. These involved 45 minutes of preparation and a mini-group dynamic which culminated in beautiful dances composed of simple, profound, moving and, we would hope, effective gestures.

I was surprised by the impact of this initiative which, despite its utopian character, was evident in the positive reaction of the participants who expressed their desire to build upon their experience. The idea was also very positively received by a number of people who could not take part in the workshop, yet who had nevertheless received word of it and communicated to me their approval. I was left with the impression that this experience offered encouragement to all those who had taken the risk that day to open themselves to a new form of dialogue.

Ongoing workshops building positive relationships

This initiative was followed up by Ayelet Ranen,[4] a rhythm dance therapist in Israel, who wrote the following account.

Building relationships in Israel

I organize Primitive Expression workshops in Israel in diverse situations and with a variety of participants:

- a school in Tel Aviv in a difficult region, lived in by Jews, Arabs and African refugees working illegally;
- workshops with social workers with mixed Arab-Jewish, and religious-non-religious, groups; and
- two workshops in the high school of Um El Faheme, an Arab town in which many children do not speak Hebrew.

What always strikes me in the workshops with participants from very different milieus, belonging to groups in serious conflict, is the ability of common rhythm to create a feeling of togetherness, opening the possibility of a dialogue in places where this does not normally take place. If in Israel everyone is well versed in equality and knows how to speak of it, if each of us has learned that under the masks which divide us we stand together, our current context demonstrates to us that it does not suffice to know this in a theoretical way. We must live it! We must feel it. As the two mothers, one Arab and the other Jewish felt it, when they found themselves together in the hospital ward next to their sick children. At such moments all prejudices disappear before our common pain.

Fortunately we can also live and feel 'the Common' in a positive and joyous experience through rhythm and a dance known to us all, that of Primitive Expression.

My workshops begin in a circle in which each participant gives his first name in rhythmic fashion. The group repeats it, making it resonate at a collective level, and measures out its beat by clapping the hands. This cultivates in less than five minutes in a sense of unity, with the clapping resembling the beating of a common heart. The group gathers together around this energy, discovering that they all resemble each other despite their differences. I then invite them to circulate in the room while greeting one another one by one through an identical sequence made of vocalized gestures. This experience reinforced the feeling of the first exercise: we can communicate and greet each other without speaking the same language. We can feel we belong to the same group even if in our everyday lives we belong to other milieus.

The rest of the session continued the work of this beginning, to which I will limit myself here. Through each exercise, the feeling that we at root resemble each other was accentuated, along with the belief that during dance we can forget our conflicts for a while.

We do not pretend to be able to resolve all conflict but this type of experience gives us hope for the future by allowing us to discover another way of seeing the other.

Clinical applications: neurological disorders

Rhythm dance therapists today engage frequently with handicapped people, in particular, people suffering from nervous disorders such as Parkinson's and Alzheimer's disease.

Rhythm dance therapy for Parkinson's disease in France

Parkinson's disease is a chronic illness of the nervous system characterised by a malfunctioning of the locomotive apparatus.[5] Sufferers experience stiffness, trembling and slowness. This illness is linked to depressive symptoms which are undoubtedly not foreign to its emergence. How are we to treat these symptoms which are both physical and psychic? Current research in progress shows that Primitive Expression is particularly effective in mitigating these symptoms.

Bellan Hospital

It is Friday, 4 June 2010, and around 20 people, men and women, afflicted with Parkinson's disease, as well as members of the association France Parkinson are in the room Trocmé on the fourth floor of the Léopold Bellan Hospital. What brings them together? The desire to take part in what, for them, constitutes a singular and novel experience: therapy through dance and rhythm. The session is conducted by me, accompanied on the drum (djembé) by Henri Samba and assisted by Hélène Banville, a psychomotor therapist, also a qualified rhythm dance therapist.

Before starting the session, Doctor Annaïk Fève, a neurologist specialising in Parkinson's, passes round some items from section III of the test UPDRS[6] for the assessing of axial and segmental motor capacity. Axial motor capacity concerns the vertical axis, the vertebral column and the trunk, whereas segmentary motor capacity concerns the limbs.[7] She highlighted certain items:

- *Item 25*: alternative rapid movements (e.g. pronation of the hands vertically or horizontally, with the greatest possible amplitude, both hands simultaneously).
- *Item 23*: tapping of the fingers (e.g. the sufferer makes a rapid, full movement with the thumb and index finger).
- *Item 24*: movement of the hands (e.g. the sufferer opens and closes the hands rapidly and with the greatest possible amplitude, each hand separately).

    The patients appear to know the test and carried it out with concentration. Movements relating to manual motor capacity are somewhat slow, yet precise.
- *Item 26*: Agility of the leg (the patient rapidly taps his heel on the ground while lifting the foot; the amplitude must be around 7.5 cm from a seated position).
- *Item 27*: rising from a chair (the patient tries to rise from a chair).

The participants, aged late 40s to 70s, presented varied physiognomies: tall, short, thin, corpulent. Not everyone performs the movements requested with the same ease. Certain are more flexible and dynamic than others. Three masculine patients of an advanced age exhibited moderate to marked trembling while at rest. These signs either did not seem present or were more discretely present among other patients.

Everyone succeeds in rising alone from their chairs and walking. Certain gaits carry the mark of age and stiffness characteristic of illness. A patient afflicted with trembling takes small steps, as do several among them, though he also seems to be afflicted by a festinating gait.[8] The patients walk straight in front of them without exchanging glances and appear a little disturbed by the narrowness of the room.

After the test, I present the atelier: the objective is to introduce the patients to an 'experience of rhythm'. I remind them in a few words that rhythm is omnipresent in nature and innate to the human body. The rhythmic gesture of dance is a stimulant which resonates with vital rhythms, and is a 'natural' regulator of all biological systems, including the nervous system which is principally involved in Parkinson's disease. I remind them also that the discovery of the benefits of rhythm have been known since the Middle Ages and even further back. The dance of Saint-Guy is an example of traditional dance therapy using rhythm to regulate the disorder following widespread cholera outbreaks during the Middle Ages. I add that the goal of the session is to allow them to benefit from the double role, both stimulating and regulatory, of rhythm. I explain that the rhythmic technique employed here, Primitive Expression, is inspired by such traditional practices, and is marked out by its strong dynamising power. Gestures are rhythmic, repetitive, recreated anew each time by participants according to a precise tempo which, unconsciously, resonates with their own internal biological, vital rhythms. This pulsation, created by the vibration of the skin of the drum struck by the musician, is absorbed by the entire body. It 'enters into us' as one participant would later say.

The first stage of the session is to awaken the corporeal memory of rhythm, present in each individual, and which we rediscover in music and songs. The participants are therefore invited to propose a well-known song which the group sings while clapping their hands. The success of this action bears witness to an unconscious rhythmic knowledge present in all humans, whether sick or not. They clap the rhythm with gusto while singing the famous popular song, 'Alouette, gentille alouette, alouette, je te plumerai . . .'. Then the percussionist, Henri Samba, begins to accompany them rhythmically with his drum. All patients follow its rhythm and therefore the same rhythm. The tempo is progressively accelerated, and the patients follow this ever-more-rapid cadence which completes in a 'stop', a ceasing of movement and silence, followed by an inspection of the body and the increase in energy which circulates through it.

The second stage solicits the body in its entirety, from lower to upper body parts, voice and movements. The patients stand in a circle, listening to the rhythm of the drum. They acknowledge it first through the regular flexion of the knees, then by walking on the spot. Hand clapping is in turn added to this rhythm marked out by the feet. The patients are then invited by the percussionist Henri Samba to begin certain movements back and forth: to advance four steps for four beats, then remain on the spot for four beats; then to retreat four steps for four beats and finally to remain on the spot for four beats. This sequence is repeated twice. The voice is then added to the marched sequences: 'Ah ah ah ah', one phoneme for each beat. They continue to clap their hands to the beat, while standing still. We note a strong vocal participation and a high level of dynamism; participants are smiling.

The third stage: the group is split in two. Each 'tribe' decides on a name and a common gesture. The first group decides that they are the 'bankers', whose gesture is an avid movement of the hand signifying that they expect something of the other, implicitly money, since they are bankers. Their hand is stretched out, palm held high, accompanied by the onomatopoeia 'Ah' repeated four times to constitute a sequence of four beats. The second group chooses to be the 'idiots'. They raise their arms to the sky and lower them with a movement of the shoulder. This sequence executed over two beats is reproduced twice and accompanied by 'oh oh! oh oh !'. The group of 'bankers' begin the sequence to which the 'idiots' respond, before the 'bankers' repeat their sequence to form a non-verbal dialogue.

The participants circulate around the room, exchanging their reciprocal gestures. I underline the importance of executing the gesture expressively, so that the gesture may take on meaning.

The fourth step consists of creating a collective choreography on the theme of an animal. Some ideas are considered. We hear some speak of a monkey, yet it is ultimately a bear which is chosen. Several patients propose sequences, and the group selects four of them. First, the bear walks four steps, arms bent and back slightly arched while uttering 'ohoh, ohoh, ohoh, ohoh'; then with the hands in front of the chest shakes the digits of the paws 'éhéhéhéhéhé'; finally, he eats the honey, which involves an oscillating movement of the hands towards the mouth while following the beat. In the fourth sequence, he crushes a bee with his right foot 'éh éh éh éh éh éh'! This choreography created by patients with assistance of the therapists is repeated several times, to the accompaniment of percussion whose rhythm is progressively accelerated. Faces are lit up and there is a clear mounting of enthusiasm.

The fifth stage involves movement in space, crossing from one side of the room to the other. Two groups face each other, one at each side of the room. They move back and forth, executing a simple walk to the rhythm. This exercise is well realised on the whole, yet the patients walk without firm posture and without presenting themselves to the other participants. Backs are arched, gazes to the ground, and there is little interaction. We invite them to walk in four time while holding their arms high and uttering a 'ha' followed by four beats without doing anything.

After they have mastered this sequence, we propose some variants. They then make a movement of the arms towards the ground as if throwing something down to four beats, to the right, to the left, to the right and to the left once again, followed by four beats without doing anything. Certain people at first make very weak gestures which are timid and imprecise. Yet, following the repetition of this alternating of two sequences of four beats the gestures become progressively more expansive, taking on form and assurance.

The sixth stage harnesses alternating pairs of movements with the objective of fortifying the link between participants. An antiphonic structure in canon is set up: one group raised their arms high then brings them low, while the other group does the opposite. The two groups then vocalise in alternation, creating an antiphonic structure of call–reply. Hélène proposes a sequence of two movements to be executed in alternation. First, a movement of the arm in front, parallel to the ground, fist closed in 'martial' fashion; then lateral undulations of the pelvis in a movement of the 'vahiné' type accompanied by the arms. The two groups carry out the movements at first in unison, then alternately. A great enthusiasm is evident on the behalf of all involved, and one of the participants normally inflicted with a strong trembling of the hands cries: 'I no longer tremble!' Among some patients, certain warrior-like gestures remain weak and inhibited: the arms slack, the movement under-developed, the elbows frozen in place. Yet, overall, the gestures manifest intensity and precision, and we note indeed a very beautiful swaying motion executed by a man of advanced age who makes a sharp and fluid motion of the pelvis. Each group proposes a gesture in relation to the theme. In the tribe of Hélène, a tall and somewhat corpulent man proposes the gesture of looking into the distance with one hand shielding the eyes. The other tribe decided to act as apes. The images are played out over a number of sequences to four beats in alternation: four beats for one sequence, then four beats for the next.

The seventh stage represents a synthesis of all that has preceded: time (rhythm); space (movement), energy (repetition), expression (symbolic gesture) in a pleasant choreographic creation where some play the role of 'warriors' and others 'princesses'. Each tribe decides on their own choreography. For the warriors, the gestures are of a 'Cubist' character: angular, geometric and accompanied by 'war chants'. The princesses employ movements of the pelvis, following the request of the doctor who wishes to observe axial motor functioning. The singing of princesses was to be 'enchanting', charming. A tribe carries out its dance, then the other tribe responds with its own, and so on. The sequences are alternated, each group repeating their own which permits the participants to enter all the more into their roles. The function of the repetitive gesture is to go a little further each time in terms of action, energy and expression. Thus the princesses try progressively harder to seduce the warriors who, for their part, tried each time to appear more fearful and to impress the princesses. A very fat man makes a humorous remark on the choreography of the princesses which he is to carry out. Yet when asked whether he would like to change tribe, he replies that he is delighted to be able to dance like a princess.

The tribes then reverse their roles in the dance, allowing them to act out different identities with flexibility.

Throughout the session I (discretely) encourage the participants. I am careful to make sure that they do not become too tired and regularly suggests small pauses for breath and a glass of water, though without sitting down since muscular blockages could prevent the participants from standing up again. During the pauses, the patients crowd around the djembé. One very enthusiastic participant loudly remarks to Henri Samba: 'The sound rebounded between us and within us, it is extraordinary.'

The closing ritual: the dance is repeated in a circle and organised this time by a movement into and out of the circle, forward and backward in sagittal formation. While in motion, the circle is divided into four sub-groups: each one is given their 'score' to play and sing for four beats. The ensemble create a polyphony and the participants circulate around the room, recognising each other as belonging or not belonging to their sub-group, calling and replying to each other, while striving to follow their own score to preserve the harmony of the ensemble. The session ends with a free dance where participants improvise to a rhythm with much enthusiasm evident.

The medical review of the dancer-patients takes the form of a UPDRS which appears now more fluid. The movements of the hands and fingers are executed more rapidly. The patients then surprise the team by executing spontaneously a perfectly synchronous collective rhythm while rising from the chairs for Item 27 (rising from the chair), investing thus a medical examination with improvisation and creativity.

Results

The patients' enthusiastic attitude contributes enormously to the warm, convivial and festive atmosphere of this activity at the Bellan Hospital. Among the benefits, the following have been observed:

- the effort involved in the activities of the session has aided them in their problems related to muscular hypertonia, stiffness being a typical symptom of Parkinson's disease. The mobilisation of different parts of the body has played a positive role in terms of flexibility, ease of movement and the ability to take pleasure in movement; and
- the pleasure visible on their faces, in the dynamism of the body in movement, in their ever more frequent interactions, in their complicity and in the joyous glances exchanged across the room appears increased. Pleasure is important for the sick, because it allows the secretion of dopamine, essential for the nervous metabolism.

The decision was taken to carry out other sessions to enable us to confirm the effects of rhythm on associated troubles, such as depression, adding to the dynamising effect a psychic dimension which is particularly valuable in this pathology.

Hélène Banville made observations over a period of eight months, conducting research on the effectiveness of Primitive Expression. She focused on six people suffering from Parkinson's disease who regularly attended sessions. She assessed outcomes in the areas of dance, energy and social bonding according to the following criteria:

- pleasure taken in the dance (in terms of the energy of gestures, investment of the body in the movement, corporeal and facial expressions of joy);
- increase in vital *élan* (the sensation of energy, reawakening of desire, reduction of apathy and an improvement of neuro-vegetative problems linked to the depression frequently associated with Parkinson's disease); and
- the development of social bonding and a feeling of belonging to the group (exchanges and interactions).

Techniques of evaluation used were the observation grille, the video and questionnaires:

- an observation grille permitted us to take note each week of the attitudes of the body, the quality of movement, the expressions of the face, energy, interactions, and so on;

176 *The therapeutic process*

- recordings were taken at two different stages, the start of the academic year (December) and at the end (May), to assess development; and
- the questionnaire focused on the benefits of the activity over the long term, in the daily lives of the Parkinson' dancers, in terms of the feeling of energy, variations in neuro-vegetative troubles, desire to leave their place of residence, variations in mood.

In a May recording, the group clearly demonstrated more energy and vitality than in December. Interactions were more numerous and greater complicity was evident. The synchrony governed by rhythm had served to forge bonds within the group which now manifested a collective spirit. The heavy tiredness of December had disappeared. The investment of the body was more significant when the gestures were addressed towards each other. The pleasure of dancing was felt not only in the investment of the body but also in the joy of the encounter, which was visible on their faces. Non-verbal communication was rich and varied, gazes and smiles testified to the warmth of the convivial interaction through dance.

The questionnaires noted an improvement in mood, the desire to meet with others and to leave their place of residence: an increase in energy (4 out of 6 after the atelier and 5 out of 6 (in the long term, six months later), desire for meeting (5 out of 6 in the short and long term), a decisive improvement in mood

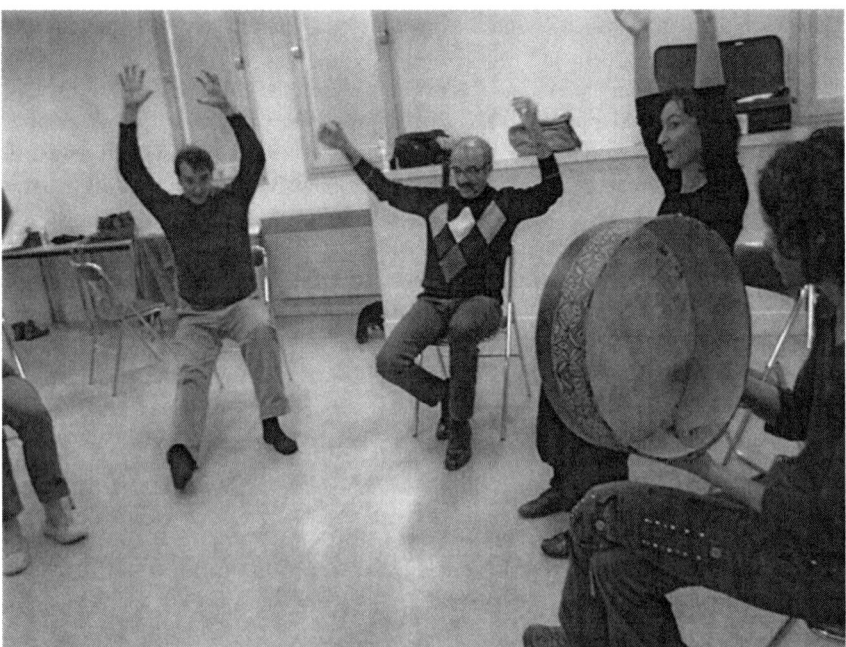

Figure 13.2 Parkinson Dance session with Svetlana Panova

Source: Photo by Ambre Serret

(6 out of 6). However, we observed almost no effect on neuro-vegetative troubles (sleep and appetite).

Patients, despite their psychological and physical pain, are motivated to regularly attend sessions employing rhythm dance techniques on account of the pleasure generated by meeting others and sharing a moment over conviviality through dance. Participants gained a sense of corporeal well-being which created a positive feedback loop increasing energy levels and a desire for life.

Besides the weekly activity organised by the French Parkinson's Association, patients have been coming to Bellan Hospital once a month since 2003 where they have been participating in our workshop called, Parkinson's Dance, with the aim of furthering our clinical research (Figure 13.2).

Notes

1 The psychoanalytical association Insistence works on the relation between art, psycho analysis and politics and strongly encouraged the project and spread word of it through its networks (www.insistence.org).
2 A Palestinian village situated in Israel and very much engaged in the search for peace.
3 I chose the term 'accordance' to designate the spontaneous rhythmic synchronising between mother and child at the foundation of their bond.
4 See www.youtube.com/user/ExpPrimitiveIsrael.
5 Parkinson's is a chronic neurological disease which affects the central nervous system, causing a progressive decline in motor capacity. The hypertonic triad of musculature (rigidity), akinesia (decline and slowing of movement) and trembling are characteristic symptoms.
6 The UPDRS (Unify Parkinson Rationalize Scale) is the measure used for quantifying the progression of the disease and the effectiveness of its treatment. The UPDRS is organised into sections which can be employed both separately and partially.

- Part I: evaluation of mental state, behaviour, and mood;
- Part II: self-evaluation of the activities of daily life (ADLs) including speech, swallowing, handwriting, dressing, hygiene, falling, salivating, turning in bed, walking, cutting food;
- Part III: clinician-scored motor evaluation;
- Part IV: Hoehn and Yahr stating the severity of the disease; and
- Part V: Schwab and England ADL scale.

The items of section III are rated from 0 to 5: 0 being normal and 5 designating maximum disturbance. 'Analytical evaluation' signifies that the evaluation was based on clinical examination, which can take place during an 'off' period (period of decreased mobility or blockage), or during an 'on' period (period of optimal mobility, possibly with dyskinesia). Axial motor capacity and segmental motor capacity are evaluated. The cardinal signs (e.g. trembling, akinesia, rigidity) alongside trouble with walking, are all explored at this stage. Rigidity is detected through the passive mobilisation of the distal joints (e.g. wrists, ankles). When this rigidity is moderate to absent, the Froment manoeuvre should be used to gain a more precise reading. The akinesia of the upper limbs is measured either alternately, on one side then the other (tapping of the fingers, opening-closing the hands), or on both sides simultaneously (via a 'puppet-like' manoeuvre of the hands) to measure akinesia in bimanual gestures. Akinesia of the lower limbs is on the contrary measured from the base of the limbs. For all items of segmental akinesia, the patient should be asked first to attempt to carry out the requested movement with maximal precision, then, if he is successful, to accelerate and amplify the movement.

From the article by Pierre Krystkowiak (CHRU of Lille) on the website of the Algerian Society of Neurosurgery. Available at: www.sanc-dz.com/articles.fr.
7 Axial motor capacity concerns the vertical axis, the vertebral column and the trunk, whereas segmentary motor capacity concerns the limbs.
8 Festination: rapid movement with small steps, observed in those suffering from Parkinson's disease. Drawn from *Terminologie de neuropsychologie et de neurologie du comportement* (rev ed. Louise Bérubé, 1991, p. 176).
9 Oral expression: the lullaby.

Conclusion

The quality of our relationships with others is at the heart of contemporary concerns in the wake of their deterioration in a world dominated by individualism, the violence of economic and social relationships, the strain on our education systems and the weakening of our value systems.

We need to rediscover our fundamental bonds, which have suffered in recent times. The West can, of course, be proud of the separation of categories which it has achieved and which has enabled it to provide secure foundations for rational thought. It is justified in claiming the success of scientific logic, which never stops inventing technological miracles. Yet, we pay dearly today for the application of this rupture which operates at all levels: we live enclosed in a private world in which our social bonds are disappearing, creating isolation, solitude, fear and diverse pathologies; we suffer from the rupture between body and mind (too much 'head' or too much 'body'), between self and other (foreigner, mentally ill, poor, young), between generations (our alienation from the aged), between the individual and the group (disappearance of festivals, of meeting places), and between self and nature (lack of ecological respect).

How are we to address such urgent concerns? How are we to create authentic social bonds to counteract the ever-increasing isolation of individuals? How are we to create inter-psychic links to repair our broken relationship to the other, to neutralise our mortifying solitude? How are we to restore the intra-psychic link capable of crossing the gulf separating the different levels of the individual?

Is it not time to rehabilitate a tool which has already largely proven its effectiveness in repairing this link, in healing these ruptures? Rhythm is by its nature a linking agent, since it couples two elements (two movements, two dancers, two sonorous unities, etc.) by according them a shared temporality. It has for centuries structured all the forms of expression of oral cultures (e.g. music, song, lullabies, nursery rhymes, dance, poetry) to the point of being engraved in the memory of different peoples. It has indeed made a return in the culture of popular rock music, which has not stopped producing ever more strongly rhythmic offshoots (hip hop, techno, rap, etc.). To share rhythm is to make society, to care for the social link and to care for the world. We cannot conceptualise our social bond without referring to the cultural and artistic heritage which underlies it: without questioning their neglect within our societies, without affirming that these heritages call out to the world today.

Can we imagine a therapy without a spiritual dimension, one which would not seek to go beyond the level of the individual? Our research has shown us the impotence of a movement which would seek to care only for the self without regard for the Universal dimension. In rural societies, dances were judged necessary for harmony between people and for the order of the world. They celebrated the gods and the major events in the history of the community. Yet today? What of social cohesion today in our urban centres?

Dance can play a key role in helping us to locate those symbols capable of responding to the questions posed by a modernity marked by an ever-increasing deterioration of the social bonds linking individuals to one another. The message inscribed in the rhythmic structures of dance and transmitted to the dancer reveal to him that he is not alone. Nature, earth, ancestors, others, culture, sky, stars, symbols, words, the 'gods' – in short the Other, resonate in him whenever he takes part in dance.

Dance reunites the earth and sky, the animal and the sublime. It mobilises the instinctual body led by the drives and sensations, leading it toward the sacredness of life. The dancing body takes flight at the same time as it takes root. It links different worlds and the enthusiasm which it produces embodies a profound experience of non-dualism, of being interwoven with the Other. What is trance if not the discovery of belonging to the universal body?

Dance de-centres the self and re-links it to the Symbolic; this is the secret of its therapeutic power and we must take care that it is not subverted to other ends. I hope that this work has enabled the reader to better understand the conditions under which this therapeutic potential comes into effect and to distinguish it from the profusion of techniques which believe themselves therapeutic, yet which do not always offer the same level of rigour and responsibility.

One danger to watch out for is obscurantism: the lazy appropriation of ancestral practices in 'magical' fashion without questioning and recasting them by recourse to anthropology.

Yet another is over-rationalisation: the interpretation of the movement of the dancer-patient through a 'scientific' grill for reading the body. Such a process ignores the necessity of preserving at the heart of the therapeutic process the mystery of the Real: the opacity of the body, the untranslatable character of what cannot be rendered by analytical language. Only (?) the arts, music, poetry, singing and dancing bring us close to what it means to be alive.

Under the feet of the dancer unfolds the royal road towards an 'other' reality: if we respect its source, which constitutes both its charm and transformative power. Following Antonin Artaud's revolt against the psychologising of the theatre, we aspire to return dance to a more intense expression of the extraordinary, where repetition leads to surprises. There can be no art-therapy without an 'aesthetic shock', without the unexpected. To shake off inertia, somnolence and pathological repetition, we must weaken the order of the everyday and appeal to vital, social and symbolic forces. We must return to rite, reactualising myth and restore to rhythm its purification function of underlying rituals such as exorcism. This will permit us to free ourselves from the prison of psychological naturalism in which the subject suffocates under the injunction of the exaltation of the ego ('me-and-my-emotions'), reminding us that it is rather through the forgetting of the self that this transformation takes place.

Bibliography

Anzieu, Didier, *Le Moi-peau*, Paris: Dunod, 1985.
Aquilie, G. et al., *The Spectrum of Ritual*, New York, Columbia University Press, 1979.
Aristotle, *Politics*, New York: The Loeb Classical Library, 1959.
Artaud, Antonin, in *Le Théâtre et la peste* in *Œuvres*, New York: Columbia University Press, 1979.
Art et thérapie, n° 24–25, nov. 1987 and n° 98/99, février 2008.
Augé, Marc, *Génie du paganisme* Paris, Gallimard, 1982.
Barou, Jean-Pierre, *L'œil pense*, Paris: Payot, 1996.
Bastide, Roger, *Les Religions africaines au Brésil*, Paris: PUF, 1960.
Bergeret, Jean, *La Personnalité normale et pathologique*, Paris: Dunod, 1974.
Bérubé, Louise, *Terminologie de neuropsychologie et de neurologie du comportements, Les Editions de la Cheneliere*, Montreal, 1991.
Blacking, John, *Le Sens musical*, Paris: Minuit, 1980.
Boas, Franz, *L'art primitif*, Paris: Adam Biro, 2003; *Primitive Art*, Primitive Arts, Oslo, H. Aschehoug 1927.
Bourcier, Paul, *Danser devant les dieux, La recherche en danse*, Paris: Chiron, 1989.
Caillois, Roger, *Les Jeux et les hommes, Idées*, Paris: Gallimard, 1967.
Changeux, Jean-Pierre, *L'Homme neuronal*, Paris: Odile Jacob, 2003 (première éd. 1983).
Clottes, Jean and Lewis-Williams, David, *Les Chamanes de la préhistoire*, Paris: Seuil, 1996.
Commenge, Béatrice, *La Danse de Nietzsche, L'infini*, Paris: Gallimard, 1988.
Cortázar, Julio, *Les Armes secrètes*, Paris: Gallimard, 1978.
Damasio, Antonio, *L'Erreur de Descartes: la raison des émotions*, Paris: Odile Jacob, 1995.
Damasio, Antonio, *Spinoza avait raison*, Paris: Odile Jacob, 2003.
Danse-thérapie, n°1, La recherche en danse, 1994.
Daraki, Maria, *Une Religiosité sans Dieu*, Paris: Éd. La Découverte, 1989.
Daraki, Maria, *Dionysos et la déesse Terre*, Paris: Flammarion, 1994.
Darrault-Harris, Ivan and Klein, Jean-Pierre, *Pour une psychiatrie de l'ellipse*, Paris: PUF, 1993.
De Certeau, Michel, *La Possession de Loudun*, Paris: Julliard, 1970.
De Felice, Philippe, *L'Enchantement des danses et la magie du verbe*, Paris: Albin Michel, 1957.
Dejours, Christophe, *Le Corps entre biologie et psychanalyse*, Paris: Payot, 1986.
Delavaud-Roux, Marie-Hélène, *Les Danses dionysiaques en Grèce antique*, Publications de l'université d'Aix-en-Provence, 1995.

Delavaud-Roux, Marie-Hélène, Ancient Greek dance as therapy, Panorama of Dance Therapy, 33rd Word Congress on dance research org. by CID (International Dance Council), Athens, 2012.
De Martino, Ernesto, *La Terre du remords*, Paris: Gallimard, 1966.
De Sike, Yvonne, *Les Masques*, Paris: Éd. de la Martinière, 1998.
Devereux, Georges, *Essais d'ethnopsychiatrie générale*, Paris: Gallimard, 1970.
Didier-Weill, Alain, *Invocations*, Paris: Calmann-Lévy, 1998.
Dodds, E. R., *Les Grecs et l'irrationnel*, Paris: Flammarion, 1977.
Dolto ,Françoise, *L'Image inconsciente du corps*, Paris: Seuil, 1984.
Durand, Gilbert, *Les Structures anthropologiques de l'imaginaire*, Paris: PUF, 1953.
Eliade, Mircea, *Shamanism: Archaic Techniques of Ecstasy*, Bollington Series, Princeton, NJ: Princeton University Press, 1964.
Euripides, *The Bacchanals*, New York: The Loeb Classical Library, 1912.
Freud, Sigmund, *Métapsychologie*, Paris: Gallimard: (1re éd. 1946, London).
Freud, Sigmund, *Beyond the Pleasure Principle* (trans. C. Hubback), London: International Psychoanalytical Press, 1981.
Gaetner, Rose, *Un Hôpital de jour pour enfants psychotiques et autistes*, Le Centurion, Paris: Bayard Presse, 1991.
Gallini, Clara, *La Danse de l'argia*, Paris: Verdier, 1988.
Goldwater, Robert, *Primitivism in Modern Art*, New York: Vintage Books 1966
Haag, Geneviève, 'La mère et le bébé dans les deux moitiés du corps', *Neuropsychiatrie de l'enfance et de l'adolescence*, fév.–mars, 1985, n° 2–3.
Halifax, Joan, *Les Chamans*, Paris: Seuil, 1991.
Hamayon, Roberte, 'Le jeu de la vie et la mort. . .', *Diogène* n° 158, 1992.
Hamayon, Roberte, *Jouer*, Paris: La Découverte, 2012.
Heidegger, Martin, *Heidegger Reader*, (trans J. Veith) Indiana University Press, Bloomington, IN: 2009.
Helimski, Eugeni A. and Kosterkina, Nadezhda T., 'Petites séances d'un grand chamane Nganasan' *Diogène* n° 158, 1992.
Hell, Bertrand and Collot, Edouard, *Soigner les âmes*, Paris: Dunod, 2011.
Houseman, Michael, 'Qu'est-ce qu'un rituel?' in *L'autre*, vol. 3, *La pensée sauvage*, 2002/3.
Houseman, Michael 'Vers une psychologie de la pratique rituelle' in *Critique*, Paris: Editions de Minuit, 2004/1-2 (n° 680–681).
Houseman, M. and Severi, C., *Naven ou le donner à voir, essai d'interprétation de l'action rituelle*, Paris: CNRS, Editions de la Maison des Sciences de L'homme, 1994.
Huizinga, Johan, *Homo Ludens: A Study of the Play-Element in Culture*, London: Routledge and Kegan Paul, 1949.
Huizinga, Johan, 'Homo ludens', in Hamayon Roberte, *Jouer*, Paris: éd. La Découverte, 2012.
Huxley ,Julian et al., *Le Comportement rituel chez l'homme et l'animal*, Paris: Gallimard, 1971. (first ed. Ritualization of behaviour in animals and man)
Jilek, Wolfgang, G., 'La renaissance des danses chamaniques dans les populations indiennes d'Amérique du Nord', *Revue Diogène*, n° 158, 1992.
Jousse, Marcel, *Anthropologie du geste*, Paris: Gallimard, 1974.
Julien, Éric, *Le Chemin des neuf mondes*, Paris: Albin Michel, 2001.
Julien, Eric, Kogis, *Le Réveil d'une civilisation précolombienne*, Paris: Albin Michel, 2004.
Julien, Eric, Kogis, *La Mémoire des possibles*, Paris: Actes Sud, 2011.

Jung, Carl Gustav, *Psychologie de l'inconscient*, Paris: Le livre de poche, 1952, 1986, 1989, 1993.
Jung, Carl Gustav, *Ma vie*, Paris: Gallimard, 1973 (première édition 1961).
Jung, Carl Gustav, *Memories, Dreams, Reflections* (trans. R.C. Winston), 1973, New York: Vintage Books, 1989.
Klein, Melanie, *Contributions to Psycho-Analysis*, London: The Hogarth Press, 1950.
Klein, Melanie, *Envy and Gratitude and Other Works, 1946–1963*, London: The International Psycho-Analytical Library 1975.
Lacan, Jacques, *The Seminars of Jacque Lacan, Book XI, The Four Fundamental Concepts of Psychoanalysis* (trans. A. Sheridan), New York: WW Norton and Company, 1978.
Lacan, Jacques, *The Seminars of Jacques Lacan, Book XX, Encore* (trans. B. Fink), New York: WW Norton and Company, 1998.
Le Breton, David, *Anthropologie du corps et modernité*, Paris: PUF, 1990.
Legendre, Pierre, *La Passion d'être un autre*, Paris: Seuil, 1978.
Leiris, Michel, *La Possession et ses aspects théâtraux chez les éthiopiens de Gondar*, Paris: Plon, 1958.
Leroi-Gourhan, André, *Les Religions de la préhistoire*, Paris: PUF, 1964.
Leroi-Gourhan, André, *Le Geste et la parole, Sciences d'aujourd'hui*, Paris: Albin Michel, 1985.
Lesage, Benoît, *La Danse dans le processus thérapeutique*, Paris: Érès, 2006.
Lévi-Strauss, Claude, *Structural Anthropology*, New York: Basic Books, 1963.
Lévi-Strauss, Claude, *The Savage Mind*, Chicago: University of Chicago Press, 1966.
Lévi-Strauss, Claude, *Introduction to the Work of Marcel Mauss* (trans. F. Baker), London: Routledge and Kegan Paul, 1987.
Lévi-Strauss, Claude, *The Naked Man, Mythologiques IV*, Chicago: University of Chicago Press, 1990.
Lévi-Strauss, Claude, *Structural Anthropology*, London: Routledge, 2003.
Levy-Bruhl, Lucien, *Primitive Mentality*, London: HardPress Publishing, 2013 (Paris: Alcan, 1922).
Lollo, P., 'Le bonheur dans la culture', *Insistance* n° 3, 2007.
Loux, Françoise, *Le Corps dans la société traditionnelle*, Paris: Berger-Levrault, 1979.
Margariti, Alexia, 'An application of the Primitive Expression form of dance therapy in a psychiatric population', *The Arts in Psychotherapy*, 39: 95–101, Amsterdam and London: Elsevier, 2012.
Mauss, Marcel, *Introduction to the Work of Marcel Mauss* (trans. F. Baker) London: Routledge and Kegan Paul, 1987.
Mitrani, Philippe, 'Approches psychiatriques du chamanisme', *Diogène*, n° 158, 1992.
Morin, Edgar, *Le Paradigme perdu, la nature humaine*, Paris: Seuil, 1973.
Morris, Desmond, *The Naked Ape*, New York: Vintage, 2005.
Neher, A., 'Physiological exploration of unusual behavior in ceremonies involving drums', *Journal of Human Biology*, 1962.
Nietzsche, Frédéric, *The Birth of Tragedy and Other Writing*, Cambridge: Cambridge University Press, 1999.
Nietzsche, Frédéric, *Thus Spoke Zarathustra*, Harmondsworth: Penguin, 2003.
Nozaradan, Sylvie, Peretz, I., Missal, M., and Mouraux, A., Tagging the neuronal entrainment to beat and meter, *The Journal of Neuroscience* 31 (28), 10234–10240, 2011.
Pankow, Gisela, *L'Homme et sa psychose*, Paris: Aubier Montaigne, 1969.

Piaget, Jean and Inhelder, Bärbel, *La psychologie de l'enfant, Que sais-je?*, Paris: PUF, 1984.
Plato, *Laws*, translation R. G. Bury, Loeb Classical Library, London: William Heinemann, New York G.P. Putnam's Sons, 1926.
Preston, S. D., and de Waal, F.B.M. Empathy: Its Ultimate and Proximate Bases, in *Behavioral and Brain Science*, Cambridge: Cambridge University Press, 2002, pp. 25, 1–72.
Prochiantz, Alain, *La Construction du cerveau*, Paris: Hachette, 1989.
Rapoport, J., 'La biologie des obsessions', *Pour la Science*, n° 139.
Reich ,Wilhelm, *La Révolution sexuelle*, Paris: Plon, 1968 (Première édition 1932).
Revue Actuel n°136, octobre 1990.
Rizzolatti, Giacomo, *Les neurones miroirs*, 2007, Paris: Odile Jacob.
Rouget, Gilbert, *La Musique et la transe*, Paris: Gallimard, 1990.
Roustang, F., *Il Suffit d'attendre*, Paris: Odile Jacob, 2008
Rubin, William, *Primitivism in 20th Century Art: Affinity of the Tribal and the Modern*, New York: MOMA, 1984.
Ruspoli, Mario, *Lascaux*, Paris: Bordas, 1986.
Schilder, Paul, *L'Image du corps*, Paris: Gallimard, 1968.
Schott-Billmann, France, *Possession, danse et thérapie*, Sand, 1985a.
Schott-Billmann, France, *Danse, mystique et psychanalyse, La recherche en danse*, Asheville, NC: Chiron, 1985b.
Schott-Billmann, France, *Le Primitivisme en danse, La recherche en danse*, Asheville, NC: Chiron, 1989.
Schott-Billmann, France, *Le Besoin de danser*, Paris: Odile Jacob, 2001.
Schott-Billmann, France, *Le Féminin et l'amour de l'autre*, Paris: Odile Jacob, 2006.
Schott-Billmann, France, in Sarah Scoble (ed.), *Arts in Arts Therapies*, Ecarte publication (European Consortium for Arts Therapies Education)
Schott-Billmann, France, *The Space Between: the potential for change*, Plymouth: University of Plymouth Press, 2011.
Schott-Billmann, France, *Arts Therapies and the Intelligence of Feeling*, Plymouth: University of Plymouth Press, 2013.
Schott-Billmann, France, *Through the looking glass: dimensions of reflection in the arts therapies*, to be published in 2015.
Sibony, Daniel, *Le Jeu et la passe*, Paris: Seuil, 1997.
Sike, Y. de, *Les Masques*, Paris: Éd. de la Martinière, 1998.
Silesius, A., *La Rose est sans pourquoi*, Paris: Arfuyen, 1983.
Soupault, Philippe, *Terpsichore*, 1928, Paris: Éd. Papiers, 1986.
Spitz, René, *De la Naissance à la parole*, Paris: PUF, 1968.
Stern, D. N. *The Interpersonal World of the Infant: A View from Psychoanalysis and Developmental Psychology*. New York: Basic Books, 1985.
Thorpe, Edward, *Black Dance, Woodstock*, New York: The Overlook Press, 1990.
Veyne, Paul, *Les Grecs ont-ils cru à leurs mythes?*, Paris: Seuil, 1983.
Winnicott, Donald W., *Playing and Reality*, London: Routledge Classics, 2005.
Zumthor, Paul, *Introduction à la poésie orale*, Paris: Seuil, 1983.

Index

absence vs presence 112, 113–15, 118–20, 123, 127, 134, 140
adualism 64
Aegean statues 89, 90
aesthetics 5, 9, 28, 139–46
Africa: African dance 8, 35, 36, 103; Afro-American dance 15, 167; as cradle of humanity 26–7
Ajurriaguerra, Julian de 148
alternation 84–5
alternative medicine approaches 54, 101
Alzheimers disease 8
American Indians: Cunas tribe healing example 54–5, 58–9; and healing 58; Navajo sand painting 51; traditional dances 23, 48, 49
analogy 98
anal stage of development 68, 69
Anastenarides 38, 51
animals: animal body and dance 4–5; animal-human link 15–25; animal play 18; animal rituals 20–1; collective choreography based on 173; dances as simulacra of animals 23, 24–5, 49, 53; human separation from the animal kingdom 116–18, 133; mythology 52; in shamanism 44, 46
anorexics 158
anthropology: and binary opposites 109–10; and psychoanalysis x, xi–xiii, 4, 42, 56, 154, 156; and shamanism 42, 46–7, 53, 54; and the study of traditional practices x, xi–xiii, 9, 37; and symbolisation 57; and warding off malevolent imagery 66
anxiety: appeased by Primitive Expression 137; discharge of somatic anxiety via motor system 11, 18, 21, 22; rhymes and songs used to help children's 66; and the rhythmic action decoy 18
Anzieu, Didier 11, 59, 75, 90
archetypes 105–7, 110, 113, 153, 156
Argia (Sardinian spider dance) 38
Aristotle 34, 86
art: art therapy 56–7, 58, 59–60, 131–2, 133, 134, 137; cave art 28–9, 30, 42, 109, 120; dance as part of the arts xii, 9; interpretations of art 159–60; primitive arts 50–1, 139–46, 154; as ritual 23; as sublimation 137–8; as transitional activity 79
Artaud, Antonin 180
assimilation 86
association and artistic expression 99
association of ideas 98, 144
astrology 101
Atelier du geste rythmé 147
Augustine, Saint 39
Australian possession dances 36–7
Australopithecus 27
autism: and body bipolarity 94, 95; call–reply structures used to discover other 111; related to fusion 73–4, 76, 77, 81; rhythmic dance used to recalibrate foundational relation to mother 96–7
autonomy, child achieving 71, 75, 80, 82, 84, 87, 95–6, 111, 118, 122, 155

Bachic dance 34
Banville, Hélène 171, 173, 175
beat perception *see* rhythm
beauty: as ritual 23; and sublimation 138
behaviour: genetically programmed behaviour 10–12; rhythmic patterns as substitutive behaviours 12–13
belief systems 106–7
bilateralism 97–101, 103–12

bio-energy 75
bipedal motion 27, 90–1, 108
bipolar disorder 73
bipolarity 90–5
bird symbols in shamanism 44
Boas Franz 50
body: binding two sides 93–4; body image 67–71, 93–4, 134, 141, 142–3; commonality of the 166; dismembered body, fantasy of 69–70, 71, 93, 113–14, 134; memory of the 9–12, 75, 156, 172; plural body 4–5; symmetry 87–102
Bori (Nier) 36
Bosch, Hieronymus 69–70
Bourcier, Paul 30
brain 5–9
breast 69, 70–1, 78
Breton, André 57
Bwete (Gabon) 36

Caillois, Roger 20
calling: the call of the world 73, 85; call–reply structures 103–5, 107–8, 111, 116, 118–21, 126, 138, 149–50, 159, 173; and simulacra 23, 24, 55
call of the world 85
canalisation 35
Candomblé (Brazil) 35, 36
carnival dances 53
case studies: Jacques case study 144–5; Laurette case study 142–3; Melanie case study 124–6, 127; Sarah case study 134–6
castration 69, 107, 114, 122, 140
catharsis 34, 77, 140
cave art 28–9, 30, 42, 109, 120
centrifugal and centripetal drives 80, 85, 86, 94, 109, 132
Chace, Marian xi
Changeux, J.P. 4, 7
chanting see song/chant
Children, Play and Education (EJE) 19–20
Chinese possession dances 36–7
cholera 172
Chomsky, Noam 85, 110
choral dynamics 118, 149, 150, 173
Christianity 45, 50
Clottes, Jean 29, 44
codification: and arts therapy 59; of chant 48; coded movements vs improvisation 11, 143; of possession dances 35; ritual behaviour 22; of trance 64

Collart, Jean-Yves 134
collective dance: ancient roots of ix; and chant/song 48; dancing for peace 162–70; and enthusiasm 39; gestural symmetry in dance 91, 92; as part of rhythm dance therapy 150; shamanism 49; in therapy 124–5
Commengé, Béatrice 50
copying and echoing 85–6
Cortázar, Julio 82
Corybantic dance x, 37
counter-transference 77, 144, 158
coupled movements 8, 87–102, 109, 123, 149, 150
creative process, rhythm dance therapy as 151–2, 168–9
Cro-Magnon man 27–8
cross shape (of body) 89–90, 93
crystals 53
cults of possession 33–41

dance movement therapy xi
Dance of the Spirits 49
Danse Rythme Lien Social et Thérapie (DRLST) 147, 161
Daraki, Maria 87
Darrault-Harris, Ivan 57
Darwin, Charles 9, 140
death: and absence-presence 70, 113–14, 132; and binary opposites 109–10; death drives 69, 81, 109–10, 143; descent to underworld 113–14; and separation/absence of the mother 114, 122, 125; and shamanism 44, 46, 50; in the symbolic world 27
de-centered ego 126–7, 140
deconstruction 153–4, 158–9
decoys 16–17, 65, 117
defence mechanisms 22, 67, 69, 81 see also sublimation
de-fusion, therapy as 75, 77, 80, 84, 85, 87, 124–5
Deleuze, Gilles 64
delirium 33–4
delusional disorders 72–3
depression 34, 76
Descartes, René 3
Devereux, Georges 45
de Waal, F.B.M. 5
differentiation 155
Dionysian tradition 34, 44, 50, 53, 64, 100, 116, 122, 156
discharge of emotions 49

discharge of somatic anxiety via motor system 11, 18, 21, 22
dismembered body, fantasy of 69–70, 71, 93, 113–14, 134
djembé 136, 153, 165, 171
Dlo (Ivory Coast) 36
Dodds, E.R. 37
Dolto, Françoise 65, 68, 76
dopamine 7
drawing 116, 132
dreams 29, 46, 98, 156
drives 28, 34, 35, 55–6, 69–71, 77, 107, 109, 127, 131, 137, 152
DRLST (*Danse Rythme Lien Social et Therapie*) 147, 161
drugs 44, 47
drums: and call-response dialogue 111; *djembé* 136, 153; importance of drums in therapy 126; in Primitive Expression 126, 156, 174; as shamanic tool 44, 47, 64, 126; and trance 64 *see also* rhythm
DSM-IV (Diagnostic and Statistical Manual of Mental Disorders 4th edition) 72
dualist (Western) vs non-dualist cultures 3, 141
Duchamp, Marcel 138
Dunham, Katherine x–xi, 153, 167
Duplan, Herns xi
duplication 83–6
dynamic meditation 50

echo 84, 85–6, 96–7
ecstasy 7, 43, 48, 64, 65
Edelman, Gerard 8
ego, de-centred 126–7, 138
Eilade, Mircea 46
EJE (Children, Play and Education) 19–20
Eliade, Mircea 43
Elkayam, Shelley 163
emotions: emotional effects of ritual 22–4; and neuroscience 7
enkephalins 7
enthusiasm 38–41, 52, 116, 118, 123, 126, 152
epigenesis 7–8, 19, 80, 85
Eskimos 52
ethics 158–60
ethnic dance 49
ethnology 43, 141
ethology 15–25
Euripides 39, 64, 150
European possession/trance dances 37–8

exorcism 34, 35, 37, 180
exploration 11
exultation 82–3 *see also* joy
eye contact 76 *see also* gaze, importance of

faith 106
fantasy of the dismembered body 69–70, 71, 93, 113–14, 134
fascination 65–6
fathers 120–8, 133, 155–6
festivity: in early humans 27; and peasant dances 38–9; and possession 34
Fève, Annaïk 171
fire: fire dances 38; fire healers 99; mastery of 27
flight, in shamanism 44, 48, 50
folie à deux (shared delusion disorder) 73
folk dances 40, 49, 51–2
fort-da 110, 114–16, 118–20, 122–3, 126
found-created object 131–2, 151
Freud, Sigmund 3, 9, 11, 20, 26, 34, 57, 64, 81, 94, 107, 109, 114, 137, 140, 152, 154, 160
fusion 63–73, 121–2, 155

Gaetner, Rose 148
games *see* play
Gaza 19–20
gaze, importance of 76, 77, 97, 125, 142–3
genetics: ethology 15–25; genetically programmed behaviour 9–12; human programming for play 19; interiorisation 85; moulds of simulacra 107; and rituals 21; symmetry as genetic mode of behaviour 88
gesture: and archetypes 156; the being of the gesture 139–40; and call-response dialogue 119; and creativity 151; dance as ancient gestural language 4; deconstruction in Primitive Expression 154; gestural symmetry in dance 87–101, 104; ritual language 21
Gnaouas (Morocco) 36
Gnosticism 104
gods/powers: and absence-presence 126; archetypes in therapy 107; and the descent to the underworld 114; polytheistic cultures 15, 24, 36, 38, 44, 109, 180; in Primitive Expression 153; and psychoanalytical theory 34–5, 55, 60; and shamanism 15, 34, 43, 46; and

sublimation 138; and therapy 60 *see also* archetypes; religion; supernatural
good enough mother 120
Greece (Ancient): *Anastenarides* 38, 51; bird symbols in shamanism 44; Dionysian tradition 34, 44, 50, 53, 64, 100, 116, 122, 156; fire dances 38; Korybantes x, 37; Mysteries of Eleusis 121; mythological representations 52–3
group activity *see* collective dance
guided imagery 55

Haag, Geneviève 90, 93–4, 96
Haiti: vaudoo x, xi, 153; Voodoo possession rituals 35
half-beliefs 105
Halifax, Joan 44
hallucination 29, 127–8
Hamayon, Roberte 20, 24–5
hands: clenched 95, 96; hand-mouth relation 93, 96; in Laurette case study 142–3
harmonics 77, 87–8, 91, 94, 98–9
healing: the healing process 131–46; healing properties of dance x; personalisation of 54; shaman as healer 45–7, 53–60; trance of possession 35–8
heartbeat 17, 47, 64, 149, 150, 154, 167
Heidegger, Martin 141
Helimski, Eugeni A. 48
Hell, Bertrand 43
hemiplegia 94
hip-hop 40, 179
holism: holistic view of human mind-body 3–4, 100–1, 141; holistic view of universe 53–4, 63–4, 101
homeopathy 54
homeostatic regulation 13
homo erectus 27
homology 23
homophones 99
Huizinga, Johan 20
humanisation 26–30, 155, 167
Huxley, Julian 21
hypnosis 53, 65, 86, 100
hypothalamus 5–6
hysterics 69, 158

Id 69, 98 *see also* self
identification (imitation of other) 67–8
illness *see* sickness
illusion 67, 107, 117

imagination: and illusion 67; and psychosis 71; and transitional space 79; uncoupling of 105–7
imitation: in animal rituals 20; duplication in dance therapy 83–6; emotional effects of ritual 22–3; in healing 55; human-animal imitation 15–16; identification (imitation of other) 67–8; vs mimism 105; and the mother-child psychic envelope 75–6; not the same as signification 133; and play 19, 20; in shamanic dance 49
imprints 16–17
improvisation 48, 137, 143, 144, 151, 168
incandescent states 52
incest 155
individuation 127–8
Inhelder, Bärbel 64
insanity 34
Insistence 177n.1
instincts 10–12, 137, 156, 166
intelligence 6
intensity 52, 55, 82, 110, 167
intermediary space 74–8
interpretations of art 159–60
intoxication 50, 52, 64, 110–11, 123
Inuit 52
invoking drive 85, 152
Israel, dancing for peace in 162–70

Jacques case study 144–5
Janov, Arthur 75
jazz 40, 162
Jilek, Wolfgang 49
jouissance 72, 122
Jousse, Marcel 86, 97, 105
joy 7, 16, 144, 150, 151–2
Jung, Carl x, 11, 24, 34, 107

Kaloyero 53
Klein, Jean-Pierre 57
Klein, Melanie 70, 72, 73
Korybantes, dance of x, 37
Kosterkina, Nadezhda, 48

Lacan, Jacques x, 55, 57, 67, 72, 85, 89, 115–16, 120–1, 122, 123, 126, 152, 156, 159
language: bilateralism 97–101; child's attainment of 113, 122; dance as 4–5; origins of human language 27; of possession dances 35; and

psychoanalytical theory 55–6; ritualised gesture as 21; and schizophrenia 72; and shamanism 46; signifiers in 120; and symbolisation 58; universal language of dance ix–x; word confusions 99
Lascaux caves 28, 44, 109, 120
latent corporeal memory 11
laughter 45
Laurette case study 142–3
learning, brain continues to learn throughout life 7–8
Le Breton, David 4, 40
Legendre, Pierre 20
Leiris, Michael 35
Leroi-Gourhan, A. 26, 27, 109
letting go 69, 144, 150, 151, 157, 158
Lévi-Strauss, Claude 8, 42, 46, 54–5, 56, 57, 58, 59, 110, 154, 155, 156
Lévy-Bruhl, Lucien 43–4
Lewis-Williams, David 29, 44
limbic brain 6
lived movements 128
logic 98, 119
Lollo, P. 166
love: dance as an act of 119; in dancing for peace 167; and fascination 65
Lowen, Alexander 75
lucid possession 38, 39
lullabies 77, 97, 120, 160n. 1, 164–5

magic: magical effects in songs 98; magical effects of rituals 22–4, 46; magical formulas 99; and poetry 100
Mammotones 52
masks 58
massage 75
maternal decoys 17, 59, 78, 79, 105
meaning and significance 56–7, 131–4, 151, 157–8 *see also* symbolisation
Mediterranean possession dances 37–8
Melanie case study 124–6, 127
memory of the body 9–12, 75, 156, 172
meter, poetic 48
mimesis 105, 157
mimicry *see* imitation
mind-body connection 3, 5–9
mirroring 15–16
mirror neurons 5–9
mirrors in dance therapy 69
mirror stage 95, 148
Mitrani, Phillippe 43
modified states of consciousness (MSC) 29, 33, 41, 43, 45

monotheistic religions and possession 36
Moraly, Pr 163
Morin, Edgar 67
Morris, Desmond 17, 116, 117
mothers: and bipolarity of the body 95; child's identification with 67–8; creation of the psychic envelope 75–6; fascination of mother-child 66; good breast/bad breast 70–1; intermediary space between inner and outer reality 74–8; internalisation of primitive link to mother 94–5; and lullabies 97, 164; maternal decoys 17, 59, 78, 79, 105; parental functions 155–6; and psychosis 71–2; regression, as aim of therapy 76–7; and repetition 82; rhythmic dance used to recalibrate foundational relation to mother 96–7; ritualised expressions of 23–4; and role of therapist 156; separation/absence of the mother 113–15, 118–20, 122; and song 150; symmetry and the archaic relation to the mother 89; and the transitional space 77–8; and troubled body image 94; woman in labour shamanic healing example 54–5, 58–9
motor discharge 11, 18, 21, 22
murder 155
muscular sympathy 13
music, in rhythm dance therapy 149–50 *see also* rhythm; song/chant
mythology: Africa as cradle of humanity 26; in modern West 106–7; mother myths 71; and shamanism 44, 52–3, 55, 56–7; universal myths 24

narcissism 64–7, 127, 140, 156
narcissistic neurosis *see* psychosis
nature: and binary movement 100–1; natural law 155; passage from Nature to Culture 121–2; in shamanism 43–4, 52, 53–4
Navajo sand painting 51
Negro Ballet x–xi
negro dances 38
Nemo, Jacques 19
neocortex 6
neotenic species, humans as 19
neurons, and rhythm and trance 6
neuro-psychology of trance states 29
neuroscience 5–9
neurotic knots 9
neurotransmitters 7
New Age religion 42, 53

new therapies 75
Nietzsche, Frédéric 3, 28, 50, 91, 92, 100, 110, 160
Nom du Père 120, 123, 156
non-verbal language 16–18, 55–8, 163, 172

object found-created 131–2, 151
obscurantism 180
obsessives 22, 69, 158
oceanic sentiment 64
ONG internationale 147
onomatopoeia 25
opposites: and call-response dialogue 119; and differentiation 155; intoxication of opposites 110–11; pairing of opposites 107–12; playing with opposites 114, 118; and shamanism 46, 50; symmetry 87–8
oral culture ix, 97–101, 147, 148–50, 155–6
oral stage of development/oral drive 69, 127
Other: and call-response dialogue 118–21, 126; connecting with (fort-da) 118–20; connection through dance 51–2, 55, 64, 87; and gestural symmetry 95; and joy 152; Other vs other 89; and psychosis 123; rhythmic dance therapy used to recalibrate I/Other relations 96–7, 138, 140, 180; and sublimation 138; symmetrical representation in walking 92
other: becoming 33; child beginning to recognise 74, 113, 117; connection with 137, 150–1; fear of ix; Other vs other 89; therapist as 123–4
over-rationalisation 180

pacifying 137
paleontology 26–7, 42
Palestine 162–70
Panova, Svetlana 176
paranoia 72
Pardo, Eldad 163
Parkinson's disease 7, 8, 170–8
partial drives 69
paternal function 120–8, 155–6
pathological possession 33–4
peace, dancing for 162–70
peasant dances 38–9, 91
permeable body 63–4
personalisation, of healing 54
phallic signifiers 121

phallic stage of development 69
philosophy, and the separation of mind and body 3
phrasing in rhythm dance therapy 149
phylogeny 9–10, 63
Piaget, Jean 19, 64, 65, 85, 86, 113, 148
plasticity, of the brain 7–9
Plato 34, 150, 165
play: animal-human link 18–20; as basis of Primitive Expression 153–8; as call–reply pairing 107–8; child acquires perspective of the other through 114; dance recaptures harmonics of childish play 88; mother–child 74, 154–5; principles of rhythmic games 154–5; ritualised play 24–5; and shamanism 45, 57, 59; as transitional activity 79
pleasure: deculpabilising of pleasure case study 144–5; and graphical representation 117; increase in pleasure from play 115; pleasure centres (in brain) 6; and repetition 82–3; therapist leads patient to 158 *see also* joy
plural body 4–5
poetry 48, 97, 98, 99–100
polytheism: dances of possession 35–8; gods in 15, 24, 36, 38, 44, 109, 180; sickness as possession 34
Ponty, Merleau 141
popular dances: as basis of Primitive Expression 153; loss of 39–40; and therapeutic mediation 147–52
porosity 63–7
possession: and hypnosis 65; and identification 68; possession dances x, 33–41, 64, 126
prayer 22
Preston, S.D. 5
primal scream 75
primary narcissism 64–7
primates: animal-human link 15–25; drawing 116; and play 19
primitive arts 50–1, 139–46, 154
Primitive Expression: and body mastery 137; and child development 76; controlled regression 13; dancing for peace 162–70; and drums 126; and exultation 82; and the fort-da dance 118; history of x–xi; holism of 141; multi-sensorial nature of 16; and Parkinson's/Alzheimers 8; for Parkinson's Disease 170–8; participant dynamics 96–7; play as basis of 153–8;

primitive aesthetics 139–46; recordings 82; as rhythm dance therapy (RDT) 80, 152–60; in Sarah case study 135–6; as self-reconstruction 77; shamanic but non-religious 38; tapping into ancient foundation for enthusiasm 38; use of coupled movement 91; verticality in 90; vocalisations 16, 76, 80, 104, 154, 172–3
primitive man, vestiges in children 9–10
Prochiantz, Alain 9
professional dancers 69
projection 67, 72
psychiatry: ethno-psychiatry 58; and possession 33–4; and shamans 46
psychic envelope 75–6
psychic roots of illness 47
psychoanalysis: adapted pedagogy of shaman and mother 59; and anthropology x, xi–xiii, 4, 42, 56, 154, 156; and the body image 68; and the dance therapist 159–60; and the de-centering of the ego 140; and de-fusion 75; and emergence of subjectivity 104; fort-da 110, 114–16, 118–20, 122–3, 126; mama and papa 120; and meaning vs significance 57; and mythologisation 55–6; and narcissism 65; and the paternal metaphor 122; and possession 34; and projection 67; and psychosis 72; and shamanism 54–6; signifiers 120; and symbolic reorientation 35, 131; and symbolisation 154; and the transitional space 77–8
psychosis: and body bipolarity 93–4; and body image 68; call-reply structures used to discover other 111; and the fantasy of the dismembered body 69–70, 71; and the father–mother–child triangle 122–3, 124–5; and fort-da 114; and fusion 78; inner and outer reality 67; main description of 71–3; and repetition 81; rhythmic dance used to recalibrate foundational relation to mother 96–7; robotic walking 92; in Sarah case study 135–6; uncoupling of imaginary world 105; and verticality 90
purification 140, 154
Puxeddu, Vincenzo 111

quantum physics 102n. 9

rainbows 53
rain dances 23

Ranen, Ayelet 162, 163, 169
rap music 8, 13, 100, 152, 179
rationalism, excessive 3
reality, inner and outer 67, 72, 74–8, 79, 120, 122, 151–2
rebirth 75
recordings: in place of drums 126; video recording of dances 69, 82, 97, 143
reflexes 10
regression, as aim of therapy 13, 36, 76
Reich, Wilhelm 75, 77
relational, dance as 91
relaxation 66
religion: Christianity 45, 50; and ecstasy 43; monotheistic religions and possession 34; and mythology 106–7; polytheism 15, 24, 34–8, 44, 109, 180; religious rituals 22, 24; shamanism not a religion 42–3; as sublimation 137, 145; suspicion of popular dances 39–40; as transitional activity 79
repetition: and call–response dialogue 126; human ancestors worked with repetitive rhythm 27; and play 18–19, 114–15; in Primitive Expression 91–2, 143, 144, 154; repetitive gesture 8, 9, 79; repetitive vocalisations 29, 58, 80; in rhythm dance therapy 80–3; self-soothing of repetitive movements 13; in shamanism 49–52
representation, human capacity for 27, 28
repression: of dance heritage 39–40; primary repression 121–2; of shamanism 45
responsorial chant 48
resurrection 49, 50
reversibility 103, 109, 126, 152
rhythm: and the action decoy 18; African rhythmic drumming for healing 36; and autism 77; and dancing for peace 162–70; and drums as shamanic tool 47; and ecstasy 64; and the fort-da dance 118, 119; human ancestors worked with 27; liberating rhythm 114–16; and lullabies 165; and the maternal decoy 17; and the mother–child psychic envelope 75–6; and opposites 123; from oral culture 148–9; and Parkinson's 171–2; and the paternal function 124–6; and peasant dances 39; in Primitive Expression 136, 144, 153–4; and repetition in shamanic dance 52; Rhythm Dance as enthusiasm 38; rhythmic dance used to recalibrate foundational relation to mother 96–7;

rhythmic fundamentals 153; rhythmic patterns as substitutive behaviours 12–13; shared rhythm and humanisation 167; and symbolic efficacy 39; and symmetry 91; synchrony 165–6; therapeutic efficacy of rhythmic practices 58; and trance 6–7; as transitional activity 79
rhythm dance therapy (RDT) xi, 7, 147–60, 162–78
Riszolatti, Giacomo 5
rituals: in healing 54; human-animal link 20–5; in Primitive Expression 135, 156–7; and repetition 80; ritual possession ceremonies 34; shamanic dance 49; and symmetry 87
rocking/swaying: and lullabies 97, 164, 165; and the maternal decoy 17; as self-soothing 13; as symmetrical behaviour 88
rock music 13, 40, 88, 152, 160n. 1, 162, 179
Rouch, Jean x
royal road approaches 57, 153, 180
rules 20, 59
Ruspoli, Mario 30

sacrificial dances 49
Saint-Guy, dance of 172
Samba, Henri 171, 172, 174
Santeria (Cuba) 35
Sarah case study 134–6
Sardinia: *argia* 38; dance of masked man-bears 52; ritual hunt of the man-deer 25
savage thought 110
Schilder, Paul 68
schizophrenia 71, 72, 83
science 53–4, 137, 141
second world 28, 43, 60
see-saw motion 103
self: bursting away from 64; constitution of 95–6, 111, 141; de-centering of 126–7, 140, 180; forgetfulness of 152, 180; and primary narcissism 64–7; re-construction of 159; separation from other 74, 111, 113, 117
self-healing 54
self-reconstruction 77
self-soothing 13
sensorial motor discordance 13
sensory motor intelligence 86
SFDT (*Société Française de Danse-thérapie*) 147

shamanism: close relative of art therapy 134; hunter-gatherers' use of 33; neo-shamanism 53; prehistoric roots of 30; return of in the West 41; shamanic cures 53–60; shamanic dance imitates animals 15; shamanic societies x; therapeutic tools of the shaman 47–53; and trance 44–5, 160; universality of 42–4
shared delusion disorder (*folie à deux*) 73
Siberia: as root of term shaman 43; shamanic chants 48; Siberian animal ceremony 24–5
sickness: as disequilibrium 45, 47; as possession 34; possession dances 35–8; and symbolisation 56–8 *see also* healing
signifiers 120–1, 131, 133, 137, 155
Silesius, Angelus 127
simulacra: animal-human link 15–16; myths as 55; and rituals 22–3; in therapy 105–6; transitional objects as 105
social function of dance x, xi, 39–40, 49, 147, 161–70
Société Française de Danse-thérapie (SFDT) 147
soft medicine 54, 101
song/chant: choral dynamics 118, 149, 150, 173; in dancing for peace 167; lullabies 77, 97, 120, 160n. 1, 164–5; and mirroring 15–16; in Primitive Expression 16, 76, 80, 104, 149–50, 154, 172–3; responsorial chant 48; as shamanic tool 48–9
Sorcerer, The (*Trois-Frères* cave, France) 30
soul 3, 43, 47, 117, 127, 132, 141
Soupalt, Phillippe 38
South American possession dances 36
specularity 95–6
spiders, dances of x, 37–8, 66
spiritual dimension 5, 29, 43, 44–5, 180 *see also* supernatural
Spitz, René 88
split representation 154
structuring moment 151, 157
St Vitus' Dance x
sublimation 5, 137–9, 145, 152, 160, 180
Sun Dance of the Sioux 49
supernatural: dance links humans to 28–9; religious rituals 24; and shamanism 46, 48–9, 52–3; and sickness 34–5; trance of possession 33
swings, and symmetry 87–8
symbiosis 65

symbolic efficacy 39, 55–60, 104, 105, 137, 160
symbolic reorganisation 40, 131, 134–6
symbolisation 101, 113–28, 131–6, 140, 154–5, 157–8, 167–8
symmetry 87–92, 103–4, 109, 118
sympathies, world of 100–1
synchrony 165–6
syzygic coupling 109, 110

Taoism 36–7, 110
tarantellas x, 37–8, 40, 66
techno music 40, 152, 162, 179
theatre 24–5, 49, 79
therapy: as de-fusion 75, 77, 80, 84, 85, 87, 124–5; ethics 158–60; and individuation 127–8; paternal function 123–6; play as therapy 19; prehistoric roots of dance as therapy 28; retracing path from Imagination to Symbolic 122; rhythm and the action decoy 18; and rituals 22; safeguards 123–4; shamanic healing 54–6; symbolic reorganisation as goal 134; and symmetry 96–7; therapeutic efficacy of rhythmic practices 58; therapeutic possession 34–5; therapeutic role of religion 22; therapeutic tools in Primitive Expression 153–8; therapeutic tools of the shaman 47–53; therapist in rhythm dance therapy 148, 153, 158–9
third pole 123, 125, 127, 135, 159
Thrace 64
trance states: and absence-presence 126; and dance 48–50; and the disconnection of individual from universe 63; ecstatic trance and shamanism 44–5; fort-da as 126; and fusion with the universe 64; neuroscience of 6; not the same as enthusiasm 39; prehistoric roots of 29–30; in primitive dance 52; Primitive Expression as moderated trance 141, 154; and reversibility 152; shaman as master of the trance 45–7; stigmatisation of 64; trance of possession 33–4; Western fear of 152
trans-cultural dance 162–70
transference 76–7, 144, 158, 159
transitional activities 133
transitional creativity 78–80

transitional objects 78, 79, 86, 105
transitional space 77–8, 79
tribal dance 49, 51–2, 91, 139–46, 153
Trois-Frères cave, France 30, 42
Tromba (Madagascar) 36

Uca crabs 21
unconsciousness: collective unconsciousness 11; of healing 160; modified states of consciousness (MSC) 29, 33, 41, 43, 45; and music 150–1; rhythm dance therapist respects 159; unconscious desires and sickness 34, 98; unconscious stock 4 *see also* trance states
underworld, descent to 113–14
universality 11, 42–4, 180
upright, humanity becoming 26–7, 89

vaudoo x, xi, 36, 153
vaudoo, initiation rituals 22
verticality and symmetry 89–90, 91, 94
vertigo 20, 52
Veyne, Paul 106
video recording, use of 69, 82, 97, 143
Villa of Mysteries, Pompeii 121
vocalisations: in call–reply structures 111; choral dynamics 118, 149, 150, 173; harmonics of bilateralism 98–9; marking paired movements 104; pairings of sonorities 97; in Primitive Expression 16, 76, 80, 104, 154, 172–3; repetitive vocalisations 29, 58, 80 *see also* song/chant

walking 91–3, 103, 108
Wallon, Henri 65, 75, 148
Western (dualist) vs non-dualist cultures 3, 141
Winnicott, Donald 19–20, 57, 68, 77, 79, 85, 111, 120, 131, 151, 153
Witz (play on words) 57
women, as shamans 46
World Health Organization definitions 45, 147, 157

yin and yang 109–10

Zarathustra 3
Zebola (Congo) 36
Zumthor, Paul 148, 149, 151, 152

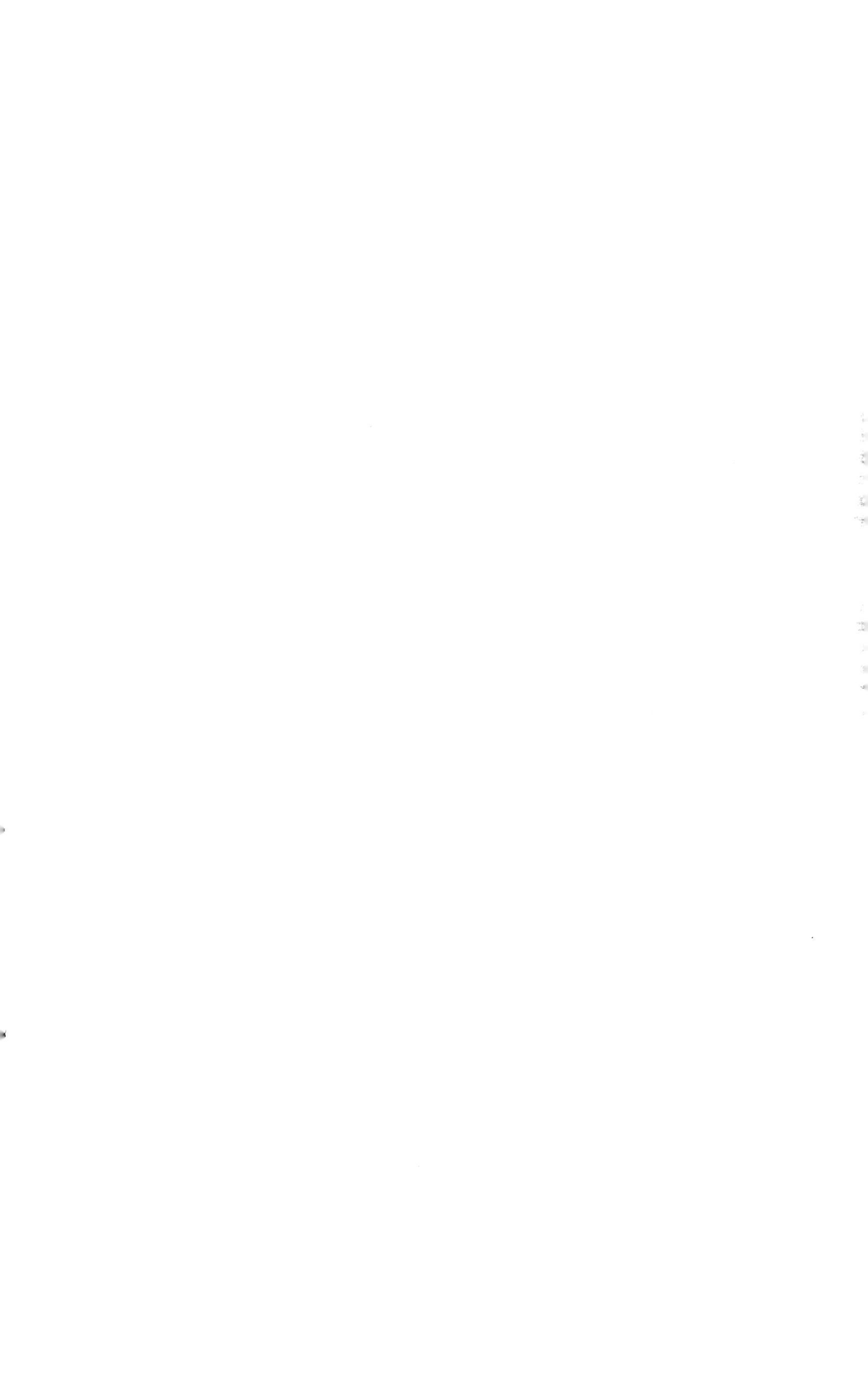